Food Chemistry

TEACHER'S GUIDE

SCIENCE AND TECHNOLOGY FOR CHILDREN™

NATIONAL SCIENCE RESOURCES CENTER
National Academy of Sciences • Smithsonian Institution
Arts and Industries Building, Room 1201
Washington, DC 20560

NSRC

The National Science Resources Center is operated by the Smithsonian Institution and the National Academy of Sciences to improve the teaching of science in the nation's schools. The NSRC collects and disseminates information about exemplary teaching resources, develops and disseminates curriculum materials, and sponsors outreach activities, specifically in the areas of leadership development and technical assistance, to help school districts develop and sustain hands-on science programs.

STC Project Supporters

National Science Foundation
Smithsonian Institution
U.S. Department of Defense
U.S. Department of Education
John D. and Catherine T. MacArthur Foundation
The Dow Chemical Company Foundation
E. I. du Pont de Nemours & Company
Amoco Foundation, Inc.
Hewlett-Packard Company
Smithsonian Institution Educational Outreach Fund
Smithsonian Women's Committee

This project was supported, in part,
by the
National Science Foundation
Opinions expressed are those of the authors
and not necessarily those of the Foundation

© 1994 by the National Academy of Sciences. All rights reserved.
03 02 01   10 9 8 7 6

ISBN 0-89278-710-4

Published by Carolina Biological Supply Company, 2700 York Road, Burlington, NC 27215.
Call toll free 1-800-334-5551.

No part of this book may be reproduced by any mechanical, photographic, or electronic process, or in the form of a phonographic recording, nor may it be stored in a retrieval system, transmitted, or otherwise copied for public or private use without permission in writing from the National Science Resources Center.

See specific instructions in the unit for photocopying.

This material is based upon work supported by the National Science Foundation under Grant No. ESI-9252947. Any opinions, findings, and conclusions or recommendations expressed in this material are those of the author(s) and do not necessarily reflect the views of the National Science Foundation.

CB787140102

♻ Printed on recycled paper.

Foreword

Since 1988, the National Science Resources Center (NSRC) has been developing Science and Technology for Children (STC), an innovative hands-on science program for children in grades one through six. The 24 units of the STC program, four for each grade level, are designed to provide all students with stimulating experiences in the life, earth, and physical sciences and technology while simultaneously developing their critical-thinking and problem-solving skills.

Sequence of STC Units

Grade	Life, Earth, and Physical Sciences and Technology			
1	Organisms	Weather	Solids and Liquids	Comparing and Measuring
2	The Life Cycle of Butterflies	Soils	Changes	Balancing and Weighing
3	Plant Growth and Development	Rocks and Minerals	Chemical Tests	Sound
4	Animal Studies	Land and Water	Electric Circuits	Motion and Design
5	Microworlds	Ecosystems	Food Chemistry	Floating and Sinking
6	Experiments with Plants	Measuring Time	Magnets and Motors	The Technology of Paper

NOTE: All STC units can be used one grade level above or below the level indicated on the chart. Grade 1 units can be used at the kindergarten level.

The STC units provide children with the opportunity to learn age-appropriate concepts and skills and to acquire scientific attitudes and habits of mind. In the primary grades, children begin their study of science by observing, measuring, and identifying properties. Then they move on through a progression of experiences that culminate in grade six with the design of controlled experiments.

Sequence of Development of Scientific Reasoning Skills

Scientific Reasoning Skills	Grades					
	1	2	3	4	5	6
Observing, Measuring, and Identifying Properties	♦	♦	♦	♦	♦	♦
Seeking Evidence Recognizing Patterns and Cycles		♦	♦	♦	♦	♦
Identifying Cause and Effect Extending the Senses				♦	♦	♦
Designing and Conducting Controlled Experiments						♦

The "Focus-Explore-Reflect-Apply" learning cycle incorporated into the STC units is based on research findings about children's learning. These findings indicate that knowledge is actively constructed by each learner and that children learn science best in a hands-on experimental environment where they can make their own discoveries. The steps of the learning cycle are as follows:

- Focus: Explore and clarify the ideas that children already have about the topic.

- Explore: Enable children to engage in hands-on explorations of the objects, organisms, and science phenomena to be investigated.

- Reflect: Encourage children to discuss their observations and to reconcile their ideas.

- Apply: Help children discuss and apply their new ideas in new situations.

STC / *Food Chemistry*

The learning cycle in STC units gives students opportunities to develop increased understanding of important scientific concepts and to develop positive attitudes toward science.

The STC units provide teachers with a variety of strategies with which to assess student learning. The STC units also offer teachers opportunities to link the teaching of science with the development of skills in mathematics, language arts, and social studies. In addition, the STC units encourage the use of cooperative learning to help students develop the valuable skill of working together.

In the extensive research and development process used with all STC units, scientists and educators, including experienced elementary school teachers, act as consultants to teacher-developers, who research, trial teach, and write the units. The process begins with the developer researching the unit's content and pedagogy. Then, before writing the unit, the developer trial teaches lessons in public school classrooms in the metropolitan Washington, D.C., area. Once a unit is written, the NSRC evaluates its effectiveness with children by field-testing it nationally in ethnically diverse urban, rural, and suburban public schools. At the field-testing stage, the assessment sections in each unit are also evaluated by the Program Evaluation and Research Group of Lesley College, located in Cambridge, Mass. The final editions of the units reflect the incorporation of teacher and student field-test feedback and of comments on accuracy and soundness from the leading scientists and science educators who serve on the STC Advisory Panel.

The STC project would not have been possible without the generous support of numerous federal agencies, private foundations, and corporations. Supporters include the National Science Foundation, the Smithsonian Institution, the U.S. Department of Defense, the U.S. Department of Education, the John D. and Catherine T. MacArthur Foundation, the Dow Chemical Company Foundation, the Amoco Foundation, Inc., E. I. du Pont de Nemours & Company, the Hewlett-Packard Company, the Smithsonian Institution Educational Outreach Fund, and the Smithsonian Women's Committee.

Acknowledgments

Food Chemistry was developed and drafted by Dorothy Goldman and Joe Griffith, and the final edition was written by Sally Goetz Shuler, Debby Deal, and Joyce Lowry Weiskopf in collaboration with the STC development, production, and evaluation teams. The unit was edited by Marilyn Fenichel and Lynn Miller and illustrated by Max-Karl Winkler and Catherine Corder. It was trial taught in the Stuart/Hobson Middle School in Washington, DC; the Chevy Chase Elementary School in Chevy Chase, MD; and the Hutchison Elementary School in Herndon, VA.

The technical review of *Food Chemistry* was conducted by:

Jesse Gregor, Professor, Food Science and Human Nutrition Department, University of Florida, Gainesville, FL

Alan Mehler, Professor, Department of Biochemistry and Molecular Science, College of Medicine, Howard University, Washington, DC

Arthur Sussman, Director, Far West Regional Consortium for Science and Mathematics, Far West Laboratory, San Francisco, CA

Catherine E. Woteki, Head, Food and Nutrition Board, Institute of Medicine, National Academy of Sciences, Washington, DC

The unit was nationally field-tested in the following school sites with the cooperation of the individuals listed:

Anchorage School District, Anchorage, AK
Coordinator: Judy Reid, Science Resource Teacher
Ed Brewer, Teacher, Inlet View Elementary
Melody McKenzie, Teacher, Williwaw Elementary School
Maureen Petrunic, Teacher, Bear Valley Elementary School

District of Columbia Public Schools, Washington, DC
Margaret Jackson, Teacher, Garrison Elementary School

Consolidated School District 54, Shaumburg, IL
Coordinator: Larry Small, Science/Health Coordinator
Marianne Zito, Teacher, Dooley Elementary School
Donna Osmanski, Teacher, Fox Elementary School

Sharon Herdegen, Teacher, Dirkson Elementary School

Unified School District 500, Kansas City, KS
Coordinator: Mary Blythe, Elementary Science Coordinator
Sue Mayberry, Teacher, Central Elementary School
Tod Pennell, Teacher, New Stanley Elementary School
Ania Johnson, Teacher, Noble Prentis Elementary School

Fall River Public Schools, Fall River, MA
Coordinator: Pam Tickle, Staff Developer
Claire Amoit, Teacher, Coughlin School
Michelle Sahady, Teacher, Belisle School
Kenneth Walker, Teacher, Greene School

Sidwell Friends School, Bethesda, MD
Michael Bass, Teacher

U.S. Department of Defense Dependents Schools
Coordinator: Richard M. Schlenker, Science Coordinator for the Pacific
Teresa Lathem, Teacher, Kinser Elementary School, Kinser, Okinawa
Dawna Ricky, Teacher, Wurtsmith Elementary School, Clark Air Force Base, The Philippines
Sigrid Straatveit, Teacher, Stearley Heights Elementary School, Clark Air Force Base, The Philippines

The NSRC also would like to thank the following individuals for their contributions to the unit:

Ann Benbow, Coordinator, Pre-High School Science Office, American Chemical Society, Washington, DC

JoAnn E. DeMaria, Teacher, Hutchison Elementary School, Herndon, VA

Charles Gale, Teacher, Chevy Chase Elementary School, Chevy Chase, MD

Richard McQueen, Science Specialist, Multnomah Education Service District, Portland, OR

Dane Penland, Chief, Special Assignments and Photography Branch, Smithsonian Institution, Washington, DC

Stuart Rudikoff, Molecular Genetics, National Institutes of Health, Bethesda, MD

David Savage, Assistant Principal, Rolling Terrace Elementary School, Montgomery County Public Schools, Rockville, MD

Terri Stover, Consumer Affairs Specialist, U.S. Food and Drug Administration, Rockville, MD

Janet Tenney, Manager of Nutrition Programs, Giant Food Inc., Landover, MD

The NSRC is indebted to all of the above individuals, who were instrumental in ensuring the scientific accuracy and pedagogical usefulness of the learning activities in this unit.

>Douglas Lapp
>Executive Director
>National Science Resources Center

STC Advisory Panel

Peter P. Afflerbach, Professor, National Reading Research Center, University of Maryland, College Park, MD

David Babcock, Director, Board of Cooperative Educational Services, Second Supervisory District, Monroe-Orleans Counties, Spencerport, NY

Judi Backman, Math/Science Coordinator, Highline Public Schools, Seattle, WA

Albert V. Baez, President, Vivamos Mejor/USA, Greenbrae, CA

Andrew R. Barron, Professor of Chemistry and Material Science, Department of Chemistry, Rice University, Houston, TX

DeAnna Banks Beane, Project Director, YouthALIVE, Association of Science-Technology Centers, Washington, DC

Audrey Champagne, Professor of Chemistry and Education, and Chair, Educational Theory and Practice, School of Education, State University of New York at Albany, Albany, NY

Sally Crissman, Faculty Member, Lower School, Shady Hill School, Cambridge, MA

Gregory Crosby, National Program Leader, U.S. Department of Agriculture Extension Service/4-H, Washington, DC

JoAnn E. DeMaria, Teacher, Hutchison Elementary School, Herndon, VA

Hubert M. Dyasi, Director, The Workshop Center, City College School of Education (The City University of New York), New York, NY

Timothy H. Goldsmith, Professor of Biology, Yale University, New Haven, CT

Patricia Jacobberger Jellison, Geologist, National Air and Space Museum, Smithsonian Institution, Washington, DC

Patricia Lauber, Author, Weston, CT

John Layman, Director, Science Teaching Center, and Professor, Departments of Education and Physics, University of Maryland, College Park, MD

Sally Love, Museum Specialist, National Museum of Natural History, Smithsonian Institution, Washington, DC

Phyllis R. Marcuccio, Associate Executive Director for Publications, National Science Teachers Association, Arlington, VA

Lynn Margulis, Distinguished University Professor, Department of Botany, University of Massachusetts, Amherst, MA

Margo A. Mastropieri, Co-Director, Mainstreaming Handicapped Students in Science Project, Purdue University, West Lafayette, IN

Richard McQueen, Teacher/Learning Manager, Alpha High School, Gresham, OR

Alan Mehler, Professor, Department of Biochemistry and Molecular Science, College of Medicine, Howard University, Washington, DC

Philip Morrison, Professor of Physics Emeritus, Massachusetts Institute of Technology, Cambridge, MA

Phylis Morrison, Educational Consultant, Cambridge, MA

Fran Nankin, Editor, *SuperScience Red*, Scholastic, New York, NY

Harold Pratt, Senior Program Officer, Development of National Science Education Standards Project, National Academy of Sciences, Washington, DC

Wayne E. Ransom, Program Director, Informal Science Education Program, National Science Foundation, Washington, DC

David Reuther, Editor-in-Chief and Senior Vice President, William Morrow Books, New York, NY

Robert Ridky, Professor, Department of Geology, University of Maryland, College Park, MD

F. James Rutherford, Chief Education Officer and Director, Project 2061, American Association for the Advancement of Science, Washington, DC

David Savage, Assistant Principal, Rolling Terrace Elementary School, Montgomery County Public Schools, Rockville, MD

Thomas E. Scruggs, Co-Director, Mainstreaming Handicapped Students in Science Project, Purdue University, West Lafayette, IN

Larry Small, Science/Health Coordinator, Schaumburg School District 54, Schaumburg, IL

Michelle Smith, Publications Director, Office of Elementary and Secondary Education, Smithsonian Institution, Washington, DC

Susan Sprague, Director of Science and Social Studies, Mesa Public Schools, Mesa, AZ

Arthur Sussman, Director, Far West Regional Consortium for Science and Mathematics, Far West Laboratory, San Francisco, CA

Emma Walton, Program Director, Presidential Awards, National Science Foundation, Washington, DC, and Past President, National Science Supervisors Association

Paul H. Williams, Director, Center for Biology Education, and Professor, Department of Plant Pathology, University of Wisconsin, Madison, WI

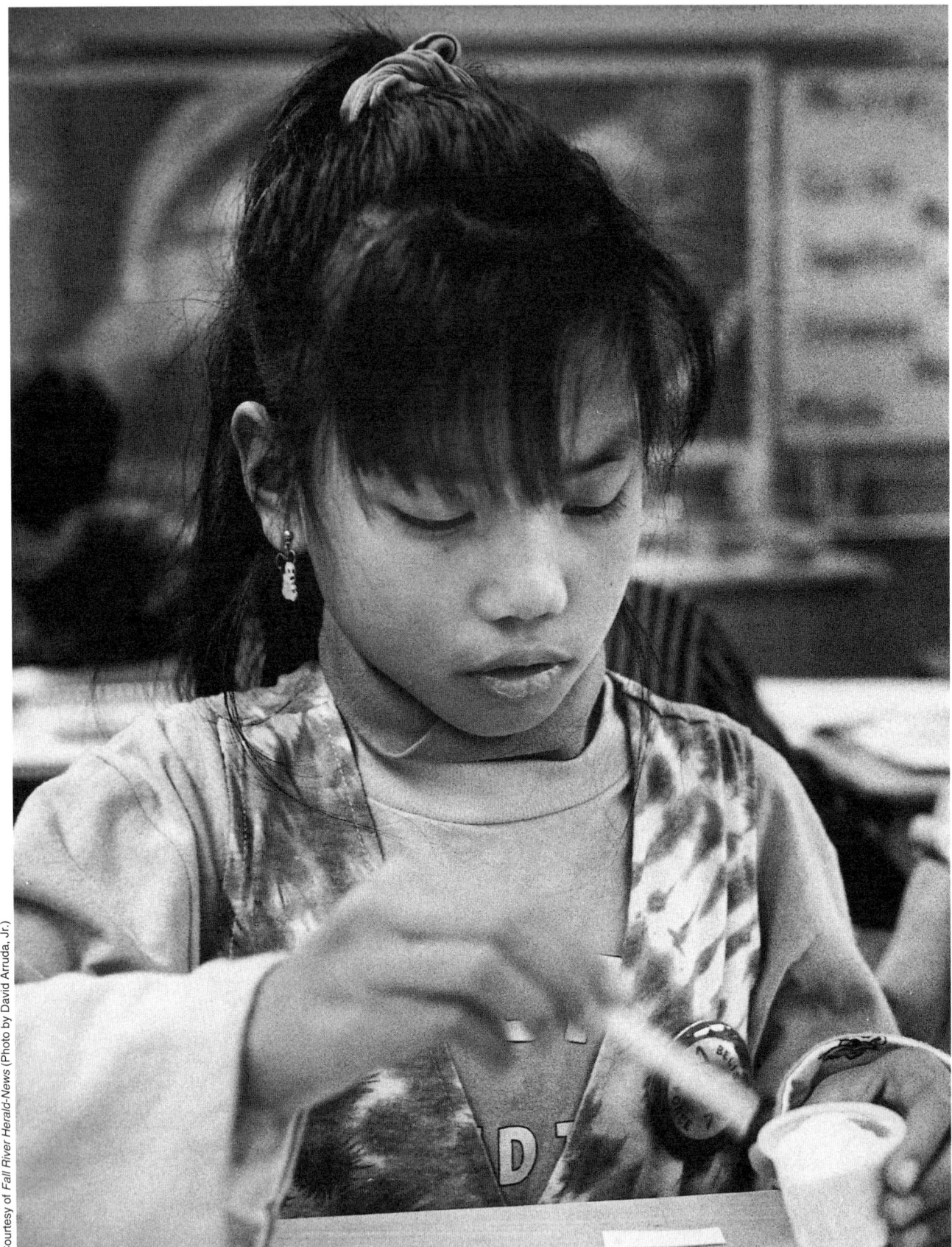
Courtesy of *Fall River Herald-News* (Photo by David Arruda, Jr.)

Contents

	Foreword	iii
	Acknowledgments	v
	Goals for *Food Chemistry*	2
	Unit Overview and Materials List	3
	Teaching *Food Chemistry*	5
Lesson 1	Thinking about Foods We Eat	15
Lesson 2	Identifying Healthy Foods: Getting Ready	23
Lesson 3	Testing Liquids for Starch	35
Lesson 4	Testing Foods for Starch	51
Lesson 5	Learning More about Starch	61
Lesson 6	Testing Liquids for Glucose	69
Lesson 7	Testing Foods for Glucose	81
Lesson 8	Learning More about Glucose	91
Lesson 9	Testing Liquids for Fats	97
Lesson 10	Testing Foods for Fats	107
Lesson 11	Learning More about Fats	113
Lesson 12	Testing Liquids for Proteins	119
Lesson 13	Testing Foods for Proteins	129
Lesson 14	Learning More about Proteins	137
Lesson 15	Examining Labels: Making the Connection	143
Lesson 16	What Is in a Marshmallow? Applying What We Have Learned	161
	Post-Unit Assessment	169
Appendix A	Final Assessments	171
Appendix B	Bibliography	175
Appendix C	Making Test Solutions and Papers	179
Appendix D	Dietary Guidelines	181

Goals for *Food Chemistry*

In this unit, students investigate the basic nutrients found in a variety of common foods. From their experiences, they are introduced to the following concepts, skills, and attitudes.

Concepts

- Foods contain starches, sugars, fats, and/or proteins.
- Specific chemical and physical tests can be used to determine whether a food contains starches, sugars (in this unit, glucose), fats, or proteins.
- Iodine can be used to test for starches, glucose test paper for glucose, brown paper for fats, and Coomassie blue for proteins.
- Varying amounts of starches, sugars (in this unit, glucose), fats, and proteins are found in foods.
- Starches and sugars are carbohydrates.
- Glucose is one kind of sugar.
- Carbohydrates, fats, proteins, water, vitamins, and minerals are nutrients.
- Nutrients are essential to human health.

Skills

- Learning to perform four chemical and physical tests to identify the presence or absence of nutrients in foods.
- Predicting the nutrient content of foods.
- Conducting independent research on nutrients.
- Observing, recording, and organizing test results.
- Interpreting a range of test results to draw conclusions about the kinds and amounts of nutrients in foods.
- Developing laboratory techniques to avoid contamination of the test samples.
- Communicating results in writing and through discussion.
- Reflecting on experiences in writing and through discussion.
- Applying previously learned concepts and skills to solve a problem.

Attitudes

- Developing an interest in investigating the nutritional content of food.
- Recognizing the importance of repeating tests to validate results.
- Recognizing that nutritional information can be used to make informed decisions about the foods we eat.

Unit Overview and Materials List

What could be more important to our lives than food?

Food Chemistry is a 16-lesson unit, designed for fifth-graders and successfully field-tested with both fourth- and fifth-graders, in which students investigate basic nutrients found in the foods they eat. Through a series of physical and chemical tests, students discover which nutrients—starches, glucose, fats, and proteins—are found in common foods. Through reading selections they also learn more about the role these nutrients play in human health and how these nutrients are related to the growth and development of their bodies. And they learn about vitamins and the fascinating history of their discovery.

Repeatedly throughout this unit, students have opportunities to gather, organize, and interpret data. They also discover that applying scientific techniques can provide them with useful information about nutrients and foods. Through predictions, discussions, and comparing results from tests, students become engaged in a science process that encourages problem solving and fosters the concept that in science, results frequently cannot be reported with "yes-or-no" answers.

Lesson 1 begins with a brainstorming session in which students share what they know about foods and what they would like to learn. In Lesson 2, students receive and set up the laboratory equipment. They also examine the foods they will be testing and practice lab techniques that help avoid contamination. After examining the class set of eight foods, each group of students decides on two other foods they will bring from home to test.

The starch test in Lessons 3, 4, and 5 introduces the testing cycle that extends through Lesson 14: first, testing five known liquids (water, corn oil, corn syrup, milk, and corn starch solution) to observe positive and negative test results; then, testing foods to identify the presence or absence of a specific nutrient; and finally, pooling class results and reading about that nutrient and its role in our health. Students repeat this cycle for each of the other nutrients in the unit: glucose, fats, and proteins.

In Lessons 6, 7, and 8, students use glucose test strips to test for glucose, and they are challenged to create their own charts or tables for recording and organizing their data. The glucose test also introduces students to the concept that chemical tests are not always clearly positive or negative. They learn to interpret results that indicate varying amounts of a nutrient.

The fat test in Lessons 9, 10, and 11 uses unglazed brown paper, presenting students with the concept that some nutrient tests are simpler than others. In Lessons 12, 13, and 14, students use Coomassie blue to test for protein. This test is more complicated than the others, requiring two steps and a developing solution. It also introduces a type of test in which the absence of change indicates the presence of the nutrient.

In Lesson 15, students examine food labels and discover that labels supply useful information about the nutrients in foods. And they read about another important nutrient—vitamins. Finally, Lesson 16 challenges students to use all the testing techniques they have learned to analyze the nutritional components of a marshmallow.

This is an exciting unit for students. They get to work with food, "do" chemistry, and gain some insight into a subject that is a part of their everyday lives. Don't be surprised if some of the questions students ask go beyond what you know or can find out. The subject is complex, there is still much research to be done on human nutrition, and people have differing opinions about what is "good" and "bad" in nutrition. No one can provide all the answers. What we can do is help students learn how to continue to find out for themselves.

Materials List

Below is a list of the materials needed for the *Food Chemistry* unit. Please note that the metric and English equivalent measurements are approximate.

- 1 *Food Chemistry* Teacher's Guide
- 15 *Food Chemistry* Student Activity Books

Equipment

- 10 resealable plastic bags, 30.5 cm × 38.1 cm (12" × 15"), for "storage bags"
- 40 resealable plastic bags, 20.3 cm × 25.4 cm (8" × 10"), for "lab bags," "food bags," and "liquids bags"
- 16 ten-section test trays
- 16 six-section test trays
- 208 blank labels, 2.5 cm × 3.8 cm (1" × 1½") for food containers and bottles
- 16 white envelopes, 9 cm × 16.5 cm (3½" × 6½")
- 32 forceps
- 16 hand lenses
- 80 plastic taster spoons (small spoons)
- 80 plastic cups, 60 ml (2 oz)
- 80 lids for 60 ml plastic cups
- 1 measuring spoon, 5 ml (1 tsp)
- 1 graduated plastic cup, 100 ml (4½ oz)
- 48 dropper bottles, 7 ml (¼ oz)
- 16 petri dishes
- 5 funnels
- 8 boxes of flat toothpicks
- 1 fine-point permanent black marker
- 1 plastic bottle with lid, 1 liter (1 qt), to mix and store developing solution

Testing Materials

- 1 iodine preparation pack (starch test):
    - 1 bottle of tincture of iodine, 30 ml (1 oz)
    - 1 amber bottle, 250 ml (½ pt)
    - 1 graduated plastic dropper
- 300 glucose test strips (glucose test)
- 50 brown paper lunch bags (fat test)
- 500 strips of Coomassie blue paper (protein test), .6 cm × 3.8 cm (¼" × 1½"), Coomassie blue .6 cm (¼") on one end
- 2 bottles of white vinegar, .47 liter (1 pt)
- 2 bottles of rubbing alcohol, .47 liter (1 pt)

Foods

- 1 box of cornstarch, 226 g (8 oz)
- 1 bottle of corn oil, .47 liter (1 pt)
- 1 bottle of corn syrup, .47 liter (1 pt)
- 1 box of quick-cooking white rice, 226 g (8 oz)
- 1 bag of white flour, .9 kg (2 lb)
- 1 bag of dried apples, 226 g (8 oz)
- 1 package of powdered egg white, 113 g (4 oz)
- 1 bag of unsalted, unshelled peanuts, 226 g (8 oz) (or a similar amount of unsalted, unshelled almonds or walnuts)
- 4 two-bar packs of granola bars (with oats and honey)
- 1 bottle of freeze-dried onions, 113 g (4 oz)
- 1 bag of coconut flakes, 226 g (8 oz)
- 1 bag of miniature marshmallows, 226 g (8 oz)
- * Fresh skim milk, 237 ml (½ pt) on each of four days
- * Newsprint or poster board and large markers
- * Overhead transparencies and pen(s)
- * Science notebooks (one per student)
- * 2 clean jars with lids for mixing solutions—from 200 ml (7 oz) to 500 ml (1 pt) is a convenient size range
- * Clear plastic tape (one roll per group of four for maximum efficiency)
- * Scissors (one per pair of students for maximum efficiency)
- * Rulers (one per pair of students for maximum efficiency)
- *13 notecards, 12.5 cm × 20.5 cm (5" × 8")
- *8 paper clips
- * Paper towels
- * Sponges
- * Plastic-lined disposal boxes or trash cans
- * Buckets, dishpans, or sinks (for washing equipment)
- * Dishwashing detergent

Note: These items are not included in the kit but are commonly available in most schools or can be brought from home. You need to be aware that the skim milk and mixing jars are essential components of Lessons 3, 6, 9, and 12.

Teaching *Food Chemistry*

The following information on unit structure, teaching strategies, materials, and assessment will help you give students the guidance they need to make the most of their hands-on experiences with this unit.

Unit Structure

How Lessons Are Organized in the Teacher's Guide: Each lesson in the *Food Chemistry* Teacher's Guide provides you with a brief overview, lesson objectives, key background information, materials list, advance preparation instructions, step-by-step procedures, and helpful management tips. Many of the lessons have recommended guidelines for assessment. Lessons also frequently indicate opportunities for curriculum integration. Look for the following icons that highlight extension ideas for math, reading, writing, oral presentations, art, and social studies.

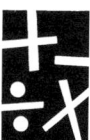 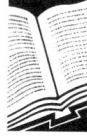 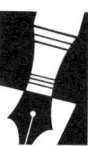

 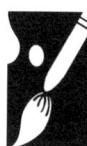 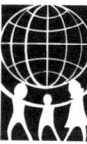

Please note that all Record Sheets and blackline masters may be copied and used in conjunction with the teaching of this unit.

Student Activity Book: The *Food Chemistry* Student Activity Book accompanies the Teacher's Guide. Written specifically for students, this activity book contains simple instructions and illustrations to help students understand how to conduct the activities in this unit. The Student Activity Book also will help students follow along with you as you guide each lesson, and it will provide guidance for students who may miss a lesson (or who do not immediately grasp certain activities or concepts). In addition to previewing each lesson in the Teacher's Guide, you may find it helpful to preview the accompanying lesson in the Student Activity Book.

The lessons in the Student Activity Book are divided into the following sections, paralleling the Teacher's Guide:

- **Think and Wonder** sketches for students a general picture of the ideas and activities of the lesson described in the **Overview and Objectives** section of the Teacher's Guide

- **Materials** is a list of the materials students and their partners or teammates will be using

- **Find Out for Yourself** flows in tandem with the steps in the **Procedure** section of the Teacher's Guide and briefly and simply walks students through the lesson's activities

- **Ideas to Explore,** which frequently echoes the **Extensions** section in the Teacher's Guide, gives students additional activities to try out or ideas to think about

Teaching Strategies

Classroom Discussion: Class discussions, effectively led by the teacher, are important vehicles for science learning. Research shows that the way questions are asked, as well as the time allowed for responses, can contribute to the quality of the discussion.

When you ask questions, think about what you want to achieve in the ensuing discussion. For example, open-ended questions, for which there is no one right answer, will encourage students to give creative and thoughtful answers. You can use other types of questions to encourage students to see specific relationships and contrasts or to help them to summarize and draw conclusions. It is good practice to mix these questions. It also is good practice always to give students "wait time" to answer; this will encourage broader participation and more thoughtful answers. You will want to monitor responses, looking for additional situations that invite students to formulate hypotheses, make generalizations, and explain how they arrived at a conclusion.

Brainstorming: Brainstorming is a whole-class exercise in which students contribute their thoughts about a particular idea or problem. When used to introduce a new science topic, it can be a stimulating and productive exercise. It also is a useful and efficient way for the teacher to find out what students know and think about a topic. As students learn the rules for brainstorming, they will become more and more adept in their participation.

To begin a brainstorming session, define for students the topics about which they will share ideas. Tell students the following rules:

- Accept all ideas without judgment.

- Do not criticize or make unnecessary comments about the contributions of others.

- Try to connect your ideas to the ideas of others.

Cooperative Learning Groups: One of the best ways to teach hands-on science is to arrange students in small groups. Materials and procedures for *Food Chemistry* are based on groups of four. There are several advantages to this organization. It provides a small forum for students to express their ideas and get feedback. It also offers pupils a chance to learn from one another by sharing ideas, discoveries, and skills. With coaching, students can develop important interpersonal skills that will serve them well in all aspects of life. As students work, they will often find it productive to talk about what they are doing, resulting in a steady hum of conversation. If you or others in the school are accustomed to a quiet room, this new, busy atmosphere may require some adjustment.

Venn Diagrams: The Venn diagram is a useful tool for sorting, classifying, and comparing information. Throughout this unit, you and your students will use Venn diagrams to discover ways in which foods are alike and different, including nutrient content.

The Venn diagrams in this unit use both two and three intersecting circles (for example, see Lesson 1, pg. 17). Information that relates to one idea is written inside one of the circles. Information about a similar yet different idea is written inside another circle. Information common to both ideas is written in the area of intersection.

Learning Centers: You can give supplemental science materials a permanent home in the classroom in a spot designated as the learning center. Students can use the center in a number of ways: as an "on your own" project center, as an observation post, as a trade-book reading nook, or simply as a place to spend unscheduled time when assignments are done. To keep interest in the center high, change the learning center or add to it often. Here are a few suggestions of items to include:

- Science trade books on food, nutrition, and famous scientists, and cookbooks with interesting appendices on nutrition (see the **Bibliography, Appendix B,** for trade book and cookbook annotations).

- A set of testing materials so that students can test other food from home or the cafeteria.

- Articles about food and nutrition collected from magazines and newspapers.

Materials

Safety Notes: This unit does not contain anything of a highly toxic nature, but common sense dictates that nothing be put in the mouth. In fact, it is good practice to tell your students that, in science, materials are never tasted. Students may also need to be reminded that certain items, such as toothpicks, forceps, and dropper bottles, are not toys and should be used only as directed.

Test Materials: Here is some additional information on the materials your class will be using in this unit.

- Rubbing alcohol: Rubbing alcohol is known to be toxic to the intestines and is intended for external use only; therefore, it is important that you monitor its use carefully. Be sure to discard the used mixture after each class (you can pour it down the sink drain). If a student accidentally ingests alcohol, call your local poison control center immediately.

- Iodine: Iodine is considered toxic when ingested in large quantities. In this unit students use iodine in a dilute solution of 0.1% that is not considered harmful, even if ingested in small quantities (2 ml). If a student accidentally ingests a larger quantity or if someone ingests any of the stronger tincture (4.4% solution) from which you prepare the test solution, call the local poison control center immediately. Also, iodine can stain paper and clothes.

To remove stains, soak the item in a mixture of vitamin C and water. One final point: Iodine is sensitive to both air and light. For this reason, it must be stored in a dark sealed container; otherwise, it will evaporate and lose its strength. (See **Appendix C** for details on preparing iodine.)

- Glucose test paper: These papers are not toxic, but they must be stored in sealed dark containers. Once the container is opened, the papers begin to lose their strength. Paper from opened containers is no longer accurate after four months. In addition, some people's skin will cause the glucose test paper to turn green. To avoid false positive results, always handle the papers with forceps.

- Coomassie blue: Biochemists routinely use this pigment to trace proteins. Coomassie blue adheres to any protein and can stain hair and skin. The strip of white filter paper containing a small quantity of Coomassie blue that is used in this unit is not considered to be harmful to human health. As a precaution, however, avoid tasting or ingesting the pigmented paper. (See **Appendix C** for details on preparing your own test papers.)

Organization of Materials: To help ensure an orderly progression through the unit, you will need to establish a system for storing and distributing materials. Being prepared is the key to success. Here are a few suggestions.

- Know which activity is scheduled and which materials will be used.

- Familiarize yourself with the materials as soon as possible. Label everything, and put on new labels if the old ones become unreadable.

- Organize your students so that they are involved in distributing and returning materials. If you have an existing network of cooperative groups, delegate the responsibility to one member of each group.

- Organize a distribution center and train your students to pick up and return supplies to that area. The most common tasks include refilling the bottles of test liquids and distributing the lab bags, bottles, and trays of food. A cafeteria-style approach works especially well when there are large numbers of items to distribute.

- Look at each lesson ahead of time. Some have specific suggestions for handling materials needed that day.

- Minimize cleanup by providing each working group with a cleanup box and a packet of paper towels. Students can put disposable materials into this box and clean off their tables at the end of each lesson.

Additional management tips are provided throughout the unit. Look for the following icon:

Assessment

Philosophy: In the Science and Technology for Children program, assessment is an ongoing, integral part of instruction. Because assessment emerges naturally from the activities in the lessons, students are assessed in the same manner in which they are taught. They may, for example, perform experiments, record their observations, or make oral presentations. Such performance-based assessments permit the examination of processes as well as of products, emphasizing what students know and can do.

The goals for learning in STC units include a number of different science concepts, skills, and attitudes; therefore, a number of different strategies for performance assessment are provided to help you assess and document your students' progress toward the goals. These strategies also will help you report to parents and appraise your own teaching. In addition, the assessments will enable your students to view their own progress, reflect on their learning, and formulate further questions for investigation and research. Figure T-1 summarizes the learning goals for this unit and where they are addressed and assessed.

Assessment Strategies: The assessment strategies in STC units fall into three categories: matched pre- and post-unit assessments, embedded assessments, and final assessments.

The first lesson of each STC unit is a *pre-unit assessment* designed to give you information about what the whole class and individual students already know about the unit's topic and what they

continued on pg. 10

Figure T-1

Food Chemistry: Goals and Assessment Strategies

Concepts	
Goals	**Assessment Strategies**
Foods contain starches, sugars, fats, and/or proteins. Lessons 1-16	Pre- and post-unit assessments and Lessons 1, 3, 6, 9, 12, 15, 16 • Class and individual Venn diagrams • Journal writing • Record sheets
Specific chemical and physical tests can be used to determine whether a food contains starches, glucose, fats, or proteins. Lessons 3-15	Lessons 3, 6, 9, 12, 15 • Record sheets • Teacher's observations of lab procedures • Class discussions
Iodine can be used to test for starches, glucose test paper for glucose, brown paper for fats, and Coomassie blue for proteins. Lessons 3-4, 6-7, 9-10, 12-13, 16	Lessons 3, 6, 9, 12, 16 • Record sheets • Teacher's observations of lab procedures • Class discussions
Varying amounts of starches, glucose, fats, and proteins are found in foods. Lessons 3-16	Lessons 3, 6, 9, 12, 15 • Journal writing • Record sheets
Starches and sugars are carbohydrates. Lessons 3-8, 15	Lessons 6, 15 • Venn diagrams • Class discussions • Oral and written presentations
Glucose is one kind of sugar. Lessons 6-8, 15	Lessons 6, 15 • Class discussions • Journal writing • Oral and written presentations
Carbohydrates, fats, proteins, water, vitamins, and minerals are nutrients. Lessons 1, 2, 5, 8, 11, 14, 15, 16	Pre- and post-unit assessments and Lessons 1, 3, 6, 9, 15, 16 • Class lists and discussions • Oral and written presentations
Nutrients are essential to human health. Lessons 1, 2, 5, 8, 11, 14, 16	Pre- and post-unit assessments and Lessons 1, 3, 6, 9, 12, 15 • Class discussions • Journal writing

Skills	
Goals	**Assessment Strategies**
Learning to perform four chemical and physical tests to identify the presence or absence of nutrients in foods. Lessons 2-14	Lessons 3, 6, 9, 12, 16 • Teacher's observations of lab procedures • Class discussions
Predicting the nutrient content of foods. Lessons 3-4, 6-7, 9-10, 12-13	Lessons 3, 6, 9, 12, 16 • Record sheets
Conducting independent research on nutrients. Lessons 2, 5, 8, 11, 14	Lessons 5, 6, 9, 12 • Journal writing • Class discussions • Oral and written presentations
Observing, recording, and organizing test results. Lessons 2-16	Lessons 3, 6, 9, 12, 16 • Record sheets • Journal writing
Interpreting a range of test results to draw conclusions about the kinds and amounts of nutrients in foods. Lessons 4-5, 7-8, 10-11, 13-14, 16	Lessons 3, 6, 9, 12, 16 • Journal writing • Class discussions
Developing laboratory techniques to avoid contamination of the test samples. Lessons 2-14	Lessons 3, 6, 12 • Teacher's observations
Communicating results in writing and through discussion. Lessons 3-16	Lessons 3, 5, 6, 9, 12 • Class discussions • Journal writing • Record sheets • Oral and written presentations
Reflecting on experiences in writing and through discussion. Lessons 4-5, 7-8, 10-11, 13-16	Lessons 3, 6, 9, 12, 16 • Journal writing
Applying previously learned concepts and skills to solve a problem. Lessons 4, 7, 10, 13, 16	Lessons 5, 6, 9, 12, 16 • Teacher's observations • Journal writing

Attitudes	
Goals	**Assessment Strategies**
Developing an interest in investigating the nutritional content of food. Lessons 1-16	Lessons 1, 16 • Teacher's observations • Student self-assessment
Recognizing the importance of repeating tests to validate results. Lessons 3-16	Lessons 3, 6, 9, 12 • Class discussions • Journal writing
Recognizing that nutritional information can be used to make informed decisions about the foods we eat. Lessons 1, 2, 5, 8, 11, 14-16	Pre- and post-unit assessments and Lessons 1, 15, 16 • Class discussions • Student self-assessment

continued from pg. 7

want to find out. It often includes a brainstorming session during which students share their thoughts about the topic through exploring one or two basic questions. In the *post-unit assessment* following the final lesson, the class revisits the pre-unit assessment questions, giving you two sets of comparable data that indicate students' growth in knowledge and skills (see Figure T-2).

Throughout a unit, assessments are woven into, or embedded, within lessons. The activities used as *embedded assessments* are indistinguishable from those in lessons. For embedded assessments, however, the teacher records information about students' learning. Whatever the assessment activity, all are intended to provide an ongoing, detailed profile of students' progress and thinking.

Opportunities for embedded assessments occur at natural points in a unit. In many STC units, the last lesson is also an assessment activity that challenges students to synthesize and apply much that they have encountered in the previous lessons. The study of each nutrient in *Food Chemistry* follows a cycle in which students first establish a positive test for the nutrient, then test common foods, and, finally, analyze and discuss their findings and conduct additional research. Specific guidelines for assessments are presented at the beginning of each nutrient cycle.

Appendix A contains several *final assessments* that can be used to document students' understanding after the unit has been completed. In these assessments, students may solve problems through the hands-on application of materials or the interpretation and organization of data. Students may also plan and carry out an experiment. On occasion, an appropriate paper-and-pencil test is included. In addition, **Appendix A** includes a self-assessment that helps students reflect on their learning. When you are selecting final assessments, consider using more than one assessment to give students with different learning styles additional opportunities to express their knowledge and skills.

Figure T-2

Sample of matched pre- and post-unit class discussion

WHAT WE KNOW ABOUT FOODS
1. Food is good.
2. Food has nutrients and vitamins and minerals in it.
3. You are supposed to eat special types to stay healthy.
4. Food can come from animals on the ground, in the air and water, including insects.
5. Food can come from plants that grow on the ground and underground.
6. Some food will make you fat.
7. Foods have different colors.
8. Some foods are not good for you.
9. Some foods can give you energy, such as bagels, candy, and eggs.

WHAT WE NOW KNOW ABOUT FOODS
1. If we don't eat a variety of foods we can't live an active life
2. Fatty foods give us energy.
3. Starchy foods give us energy.
4. Sugary foods are good for quick energy.
5. Very few foods have only one nutrient.
6. A lot of the best tasting foods have all three nutrients.
7. You can read labels to find out what is in foods.
8. Fats aren't all bad.
9. Protein comes from plants and animals.

Documenting Student Performance: In STC units, assessment is based on your recorded observations and students' work products and oral communication. All these documentation methods together will give you a comprehensive picture of each student's growth.

Teachers' *observations and anecdotal notes* often provide the most useful information about students' understanding. Because it is important to document observations used for assessment, teachers frequently keep note cards, journals, or checklists. Many lessons include guidelines to help you focus your observations. Each day, you should try to record your observations of a small group of students. By the end of the unit, you will have numerous observations for every student in your class. The blackline master on pg. 12 provides a format you may want to use or adapt for recording observations. It includes this unit's goals for science concepts and skills.

Work products, which include both what students write and what they make, indicate students' progress toward the goals of the unit. Examine students' work regularly; their written materials should be kept together in their science notebooks to document learning over the course of the unit. When students refer back to their work from previous lessons, they can reflect on their learning.

A variety of materials are produced during a unit. Record sheets—for example, written observations, drawings, graphs, tables, and charts—are an important part of all STC units. They provide evidence of each student's ability to collect, record, and process information. Students' science notebooks or journals are another type of work product. Often a rich source of information for assessment, notebooks reveal how students have organized their data and what their thoughts, ideas, and questions have been over time. In some cases, students do not write or draw well enough for their products to be used for assessment purposes, but their experiences in trying to express themselves on paper are nonetheless beneficial. Other work products might include Venn diagrams, posters, and written research reports.

Oral communication—what students say formally and informally in class and in individual sessions with you—is a particularly useful way to learn what students know. Ongoing records of class and small-group discussions should be a part of your documentation of students' learning. Interviews of your students can be used both to explore their thoughts and to diagnose their needs; patterns in students' thinking often surface, for example, when carefully formulated questions stimulate students to explain their reasoning or the steps they used in a process. The questions that students themselves ask also can be a valuable source of information about their understanding. Individual and group presentations can give you insights about the meanings your students have assigned to procedures and concepts and about their confidence in their learning; in fact, a student's verbal description of a chart, experiment, or graph is frequently more useful for assessment than the product or results. Questions posed by other students following presentations provide yet another opportunity for you to gather information.

Blackline Master
Food Chemistry: Observations of Student Performance

STUDENT'S NAME:

Concepts | Observations

- Foods contain starches, sugars, fats, and/or proteins.

- Specific chemical and physical tests can be used to determine whether a food contains starches, glucose, fats, or proteins.

- Iodine can be used to test for starches, glucose test paper for glucose, brown paper for fats, and Coomassie blue for proteins.

- Varying amounts of starches, glucose, fats, and proteins are found in foods.

- Starches and sugars are carbohydrates.

- Glucose is one kind of sugar.

- Carbohydrates, fats, proteins, water, vitamins, and minerals are nutrients.

- Nutrients are essential to human health.

Skills

- Learning to perform four chemical and physical tests to identify the presence or absence of nutrients in foods.

- Predicting the nutrient content of foods.

- Conducting independent research on nutrients.

- Observing, recording, and organizing test results.

- Interpreting a range of test results to draw conclusions about the kinds and amounts of nutrients in foods.

- Developing laboratory techniques to avoid contamination of the test samples.

- Communicating results in writing and through discussion.

- Reflecting on experiences in writing and through discussion.

- Applying previously learned concepts and skills to solve a problem.

STC / *Food Chemistry*

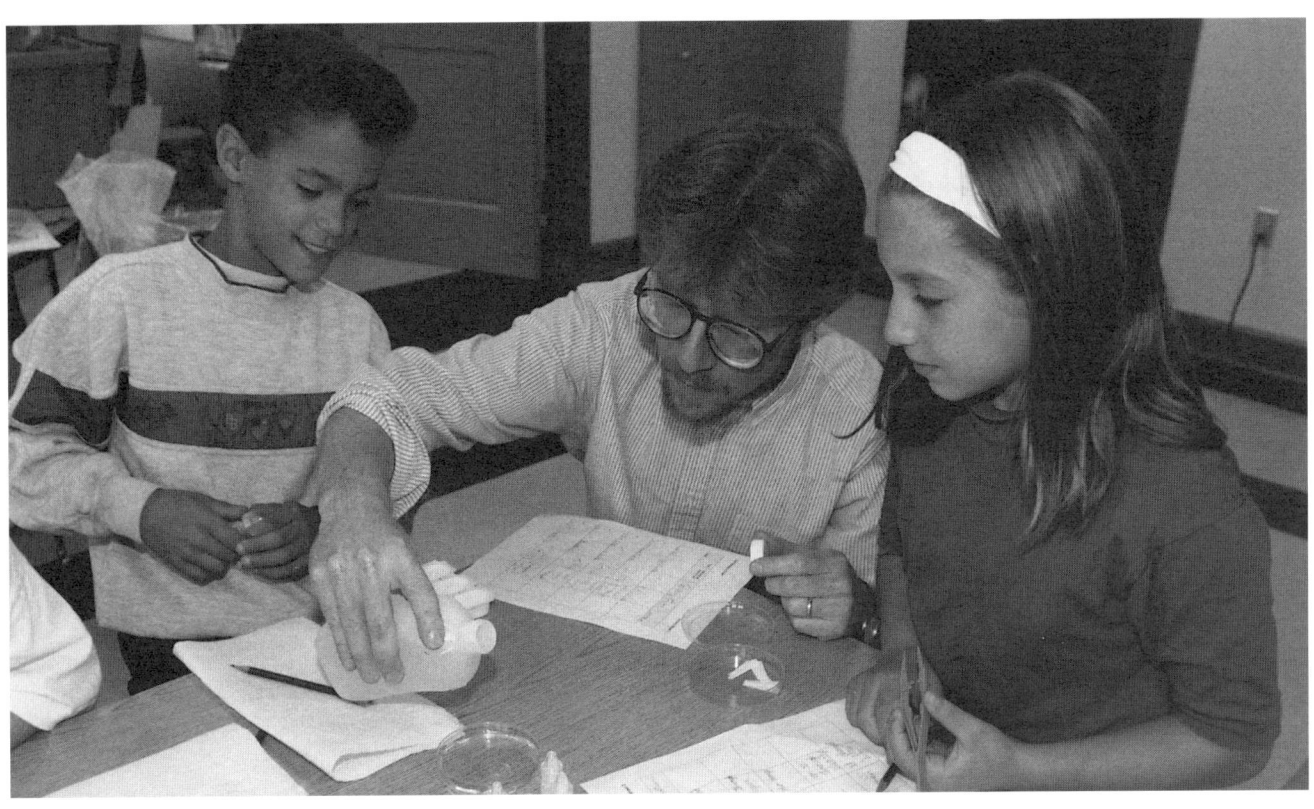

LESSON 1

Thinking about Foods We Eat

Overview and Objectives

This introductory lesson sets the stage for students to explore food and nutrition. By brainstorming what they know about foods in general and discussing foods they eat for specific meals, students begin to consider the relationship of nutrition to human health. Responses and questions in this lesson are useful as a pre-unit assessment of how students currently relate food and nutrition to their daily lives.

- Students prepare their science notebooks for record-keeping.

- Students record individually and then discuss as a group what they already know about the foods they eat and what they would like to learn.

- Working in groups, students draw upon their daily experiences with food to identify and categorize the foods they eat for breakfast, lunch, and dinner.

Background

Chemistry is the study of chemicals and how they interact. Everything is made up of chemicals, whether it exists in nature or is made by humans. We are made of chemicals. We produce chemicals, such as carbon dioxide, as part of our living processes. To live, we need to consume chemicals from the air we breathe, the water we drink, and the food we eat.

Food provides us with important chemicals called nutrients. Those needed by the body in large quantities—**water, carbohydrates, proteins,** and **fats**—are called **macronutrients**. They fill many of the body's needs, including growth, cell repair, and the provision of energy. **Micronutrients**, which the body needs in smaller quantities, include vitamins and minerals.

Carbohydrates—sugars and starches—provide mainly energy. Many foods from plants provide carbohydrates. Potatoes, rice, pasta, and breads are all rich in carbohydrates. The body changes surplus carbohydrates to fat for storage.

Our bodies need proteins for growth and repair. We get proteins from both plants and animals. Fish and the lean parts of beef, chicken, and pork are rich in proteins, as are beans and milk. Our bodies cannot store extra proteins.

Fats provide energy for the body and can be stored for long periods of time. They also cushion our organs and insulate us from the cold. Fats occur in almost all foods but are abundant in nuts, whole milk, cream, butter, seeds, eggs, and the fatty part of meats. Vegetable oils, such as those from corn and olives, are also fats.

LESSON 1

Minerals (such as calcium, iodine, and iron) are a necessary part of all cells and body fluids and enter into many of the body's physiological and structural functions. We need vitamins in only small quantities, but they play an important role. Vitamins enable the body to metabolize other nutrients it needs to grow and remain healthy. Students will learn about some specific vitamins in the **Reading Selections** beginning on pg. 150 in Lesson 15.

The **Background** sections and **Reading Selections** in ensuing lessons will reiterate some of this information in greater detail, as it pertains to each lesson. References listed in the **Bibliography** in **Appendix B** provide more in-depth information about these topics.

Note: When students share what they know about foods, someone may bring up the traditional "four food groups." This specific method of organizing foods is no longer recognized by experts as the most up-to-date. Recent information related to this area can be found in the 1991 dietary guidelines produced by the U.S. Department of Health and Human Services, U.S. Department of Agriculture, and the National Research Council (see **Appendix D** on pg. 181).

Materials

For each student
- 1 science notebook (looseleaf or folder with pockets)
- 1 **Record Sheet 1-A, Foods We Eat for Different Meals**

For every two students
- 1 *Food Chemistry* Student Activity Book

For the class
- 3 large sheets of newsprint or poster board and large marker

Preparation

1. Write each of the following titles on a sheet of newsprint or poster board:
   - "What We Know about Foods"
   - "Questions We Have about Foods"

2. On another sheet of newsprint or poster board, draw a class Venn diagram and title it "Foods We Eat for Different Meals" (see Figure 1-1).

   Note: See pg. 6 of this guide for an explanation of Venn diagrams and some suggestions for how to use them.

3. Make one copy of **Record Sheet 1-A, Foods We Eat for Different Meals** for each student.

4. Review this lesson as it is presented in the Student Activity Book. Decide when in this lesson you want to distribute the book to students.

Procedure

1. To introduce the overall goals of the *Food Chemistry* unit to the class, help students understand that they will discuss what they know about the foods they eat and what they want to find out. Then, over the next several weeks, the class will conduct a series of investigations to identify the nutrients contained in different foods. And, students will be making a number of discoveries about how the foods they eat affect their health.

Figure 1-1

Class Venn diagram

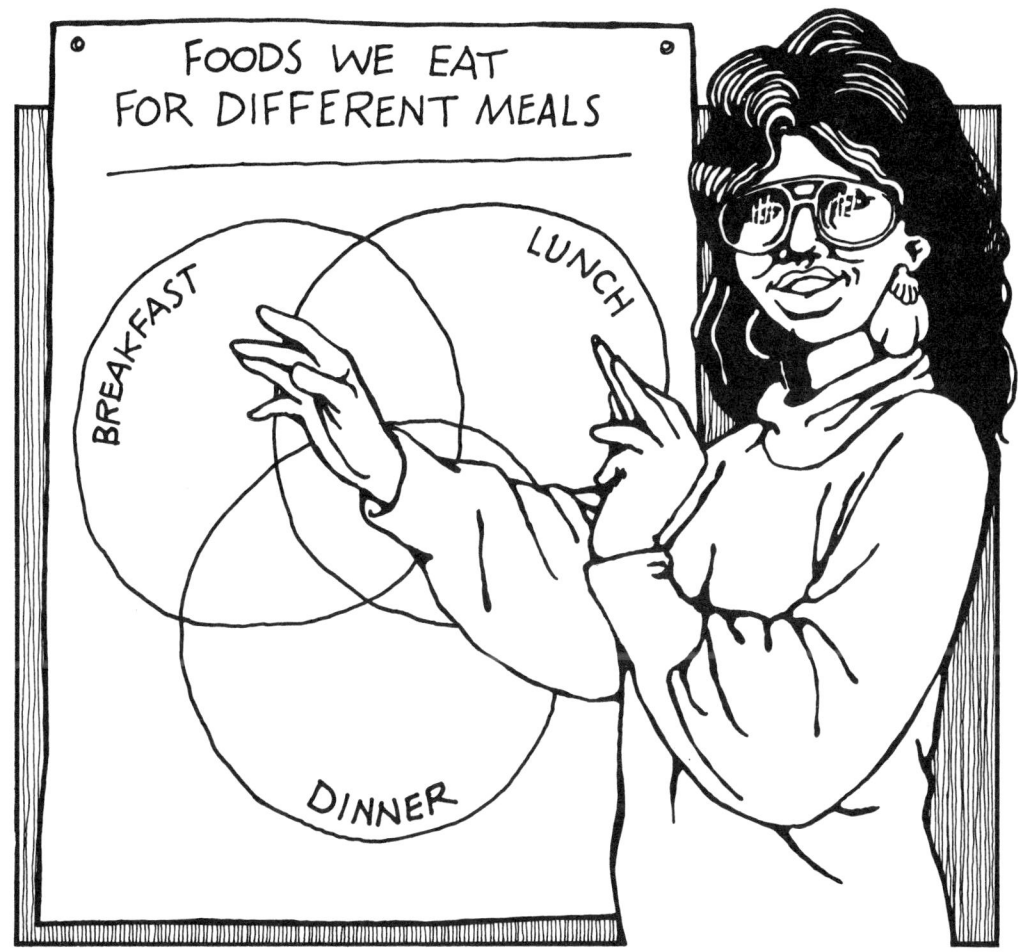

2. Next, ask students to write today's date in their science notebooks. (Point out the importance of recording the date every time they write in their notebooks throughout the unit.) As a preparation for class discussion, have them spend about five minutes on their own writing several things they know about the foods they eat.

3. Display the "What We Know about Foods" sheet and ask students to begin sharing some of the ideas they have written (see Figure 1-2 for some examples of past student responses).

4. Following this discussion, arrange students in groups of four and pass out **Record Sheet 1-A, Foods We Eat for Different Meals**. Explain that this is called a Venn diagram and briefly discuss how to record information on it.

5. Then have the groups discuss the foods they or their families, relatives, and friends eat for breakfast, lunch, and dinner. As ideas are generated, ask each student to record all of the group's ideas on his or her own copy of the Venn diagram. Also have each group choose a spokesperson to report that group's ideas to the class (see Figure 1-3).

Figure 1-2

Sample brainstorming list

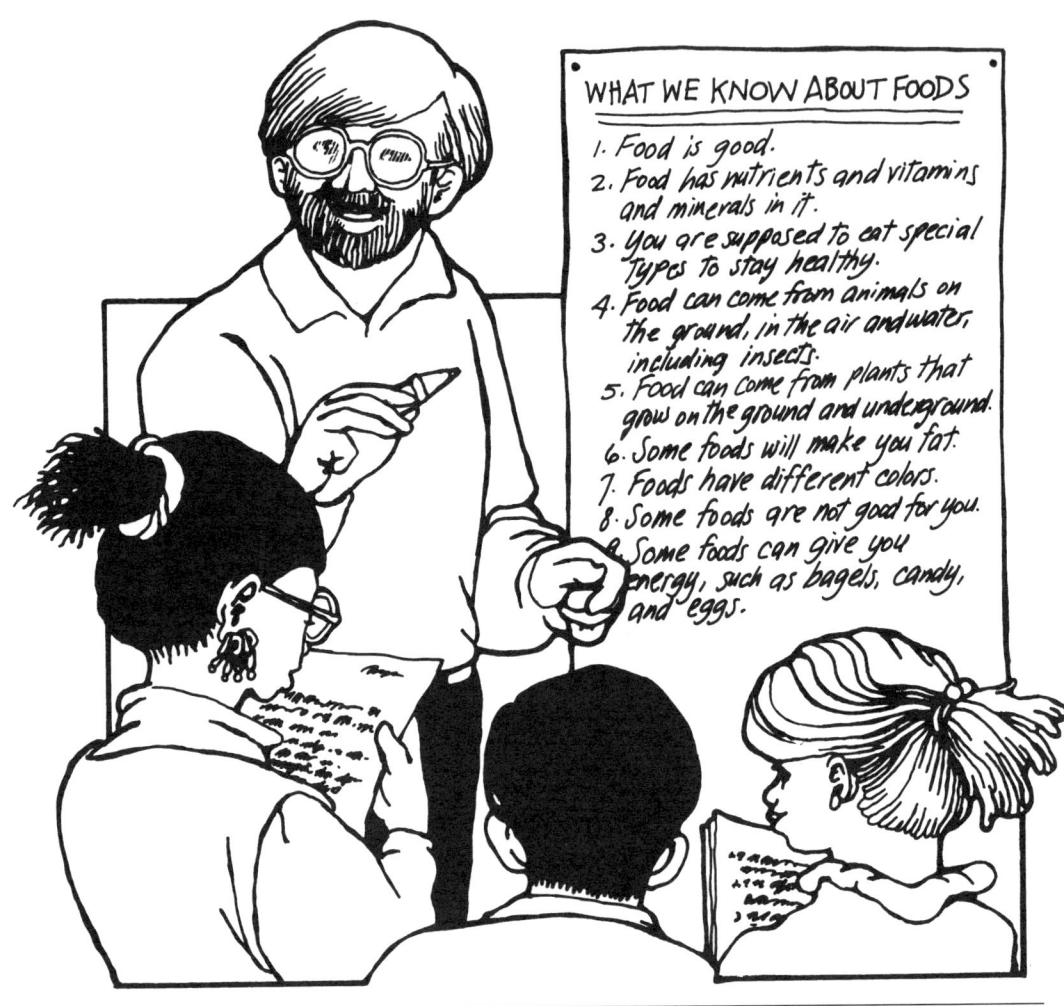

Final Activities

1. Conduct a class discussion by asking the spokesperson from each group to report that group's ideas to the class. Starting with breakfast, ask students to name several foods and record them on the class Venn diagram you prepared earlier. Then do the same for lunch and dinner. Be sure to put a check next to any "repeat" ideas to acknowledge every group's contribution.

   Note: Save the class Venn diagram of breakfast, lunch, and dinner foods to use in the next lesson.

2. Following this discussion, ask students what questions they have about food. Record these on the "Questions We Have about Foods" sheet. Keep this list up in the classroom, and encourage students to add to it throughout the unit.

Figure 1-3

Sample class Venn diagram

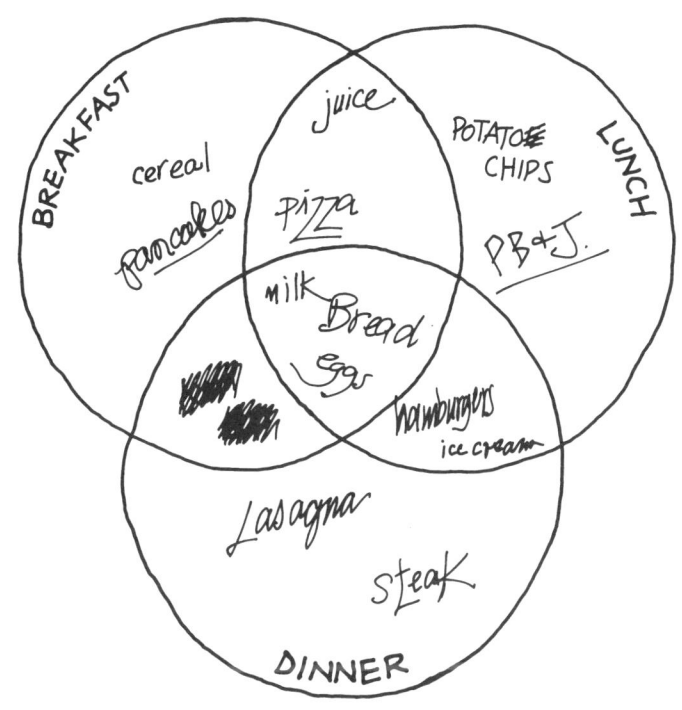

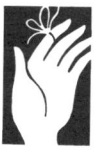

Management Tip: Starting with Lesson 2, students will be working with a set of test foods: rice, flour, dried apples, powdered egg white, peanuts, granola bar, freeze-dried onion, and coconut flakes. To prepare for that lesson, assemble one set of foods for every four students ahead of time. (You may also want to ask a student or parent volunteer to help.) See the instructions in the **Preparation** section of Lesson 2, on pg. 25.

Extensions

1. Have students do some research on what different cultures eat for breakfast, lunch, and dinner. Students can present a culture's mealtime preferences in the form of a Venn diagram similar to the one they completed in this lesson.

2. Ask students to find interesting articles about foods in newspapers and magazines and to share these articles with the class. Students may prepare oral reports or create a class bulletin board.

3. Have students make mobiles of foods for different meals.

Assessment

In the section **Teaching Food Chemistry**, on pgs. 7 to 11, you will find a detailed discussion about the assessment of students' learning. The specific goals and related assessments for this unit are summarized in Figure T-1 on pgs. 8 and 9.

In this lesson, each student's notebook entries and Venn diagram will provide an important pre-unit assessment of current knowledge about food and nutrition. This information serves as the first part of the matched pre- and post-unit assessments, which are integral to teaching the unit. The brainstorming chart is also used as a matched pre- and post-unit assessment for the class. The post-unit assessment is on pg. 169, following Lesson 16.

LESSON 1

As you read the notebook entries and Venn diagrams and as you observe class activities during this lesson, keep the following criteria in mind:

- Of the information students already have about foods, which is accurate and based on experience?
- Have students had previous experience studying foods or nutrition?
- Are their questions about specific foods or about food in general?
- Are students aware that foods contain carbohydrates, fats, proteins, vitamins, and minerals?

Throughout the unit, students will record what they are learning. By comparing these entries at different times, you will be able to assess individual growth.

Record Sheet 1-A   Name: _____

Date: _____

Foods We Eat for Different Meals

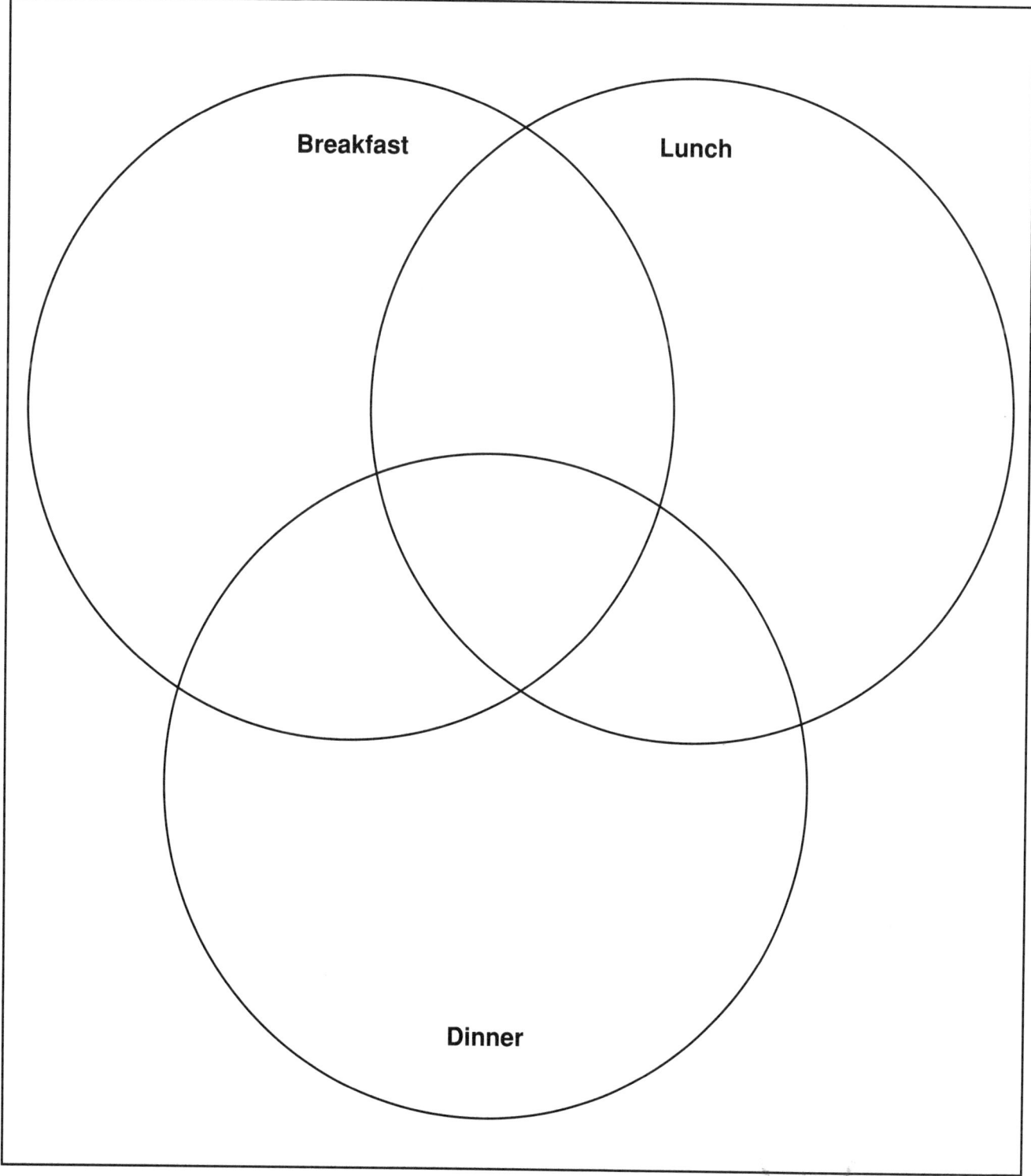

STC / *Food Chemistry*

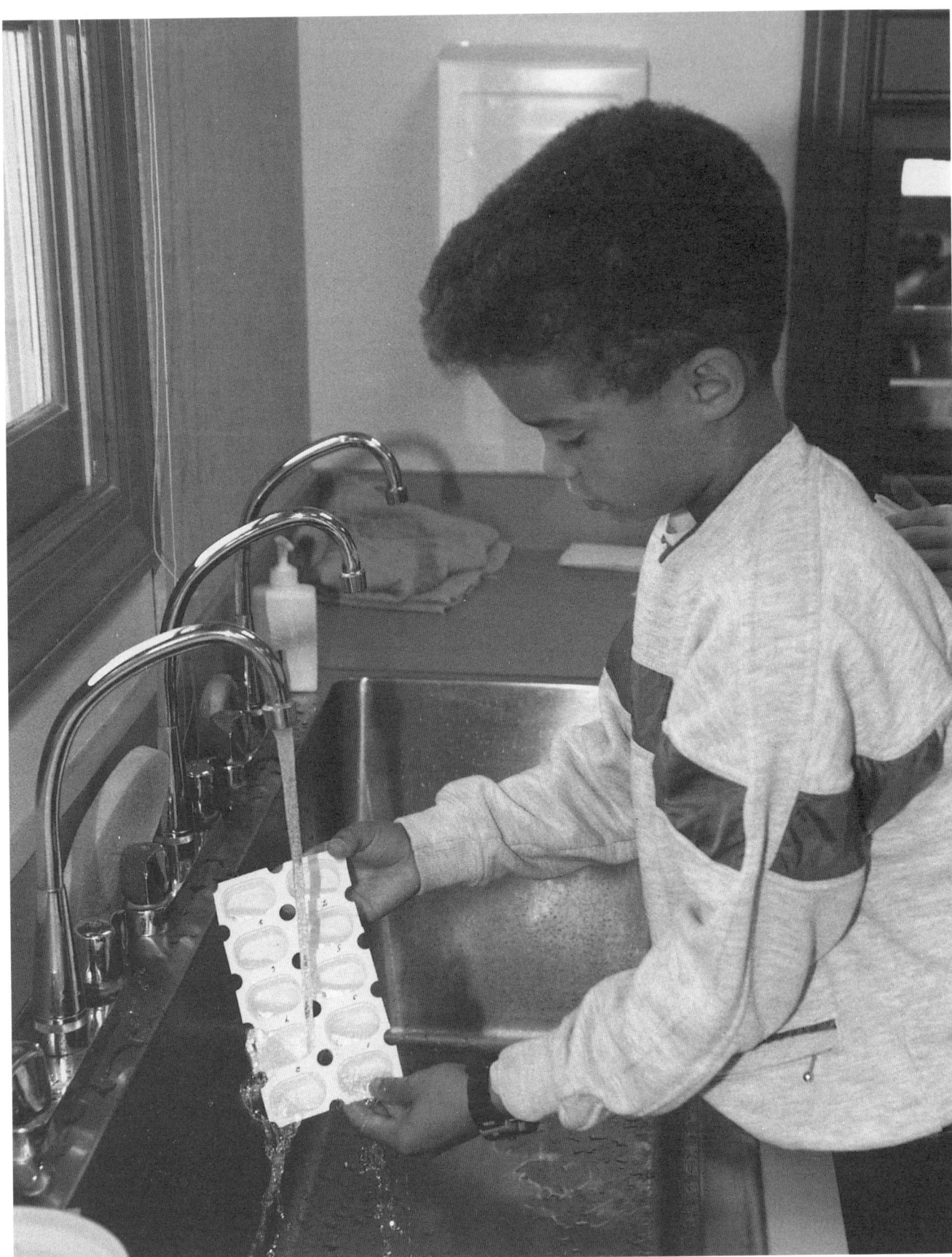

LESSON 2

Identifying Healthy Foods: Getting Ready

Overview and Objectives

In the first lesson, students shared their general ideas and questions about foods they eat. Lesson 2 elicits their current thinking about "healthy" foods and introduces scientific procedures for determining the nutrients in foods. As students observe the eight foods they will test later for starch, glucose, fat, and protein, they begin to think about why it is important to use laboratory equipment carefully.

- Students discuss why they think certain foods are "healthy," and propose ways to find out more about the contents of foods.

- Students organize the food testing equipment they will use throughout the unit, and become familiar with how they should use it to obtain accurate test results.

- Students observe the test foods and discuss their findings.

Background

How can you tell if certain foods are good for you or not? This is actually a complex problem since most foods, even so-called junk food such as candy bars and potato chips, have at least some nutritional value. It is important to keep in mind that a balanced diet is the result of three factors: what you eat, when you eat it, and what other foods you eat with it.

In this lesson, when you ask students to think about which foods are healthy, be prepared for a wide variety of responses. For example, many children may consider fruits and vegetables healthy but think of ice cream and candy as junk food. On the other hand, students are likely to disagree about whether foods such as meat, bread, and potatoes are healthy.

Remember that students' ideas are the result of personal experiences and any earlier studies of food. At this time, accept all responses and encourage students to reevaluate their ideas about the relationship of food and nutrition as they carry out their food investigations in ensuing lessons. Students will revisit their ideas about healthy foods at the end of the unit.

Also in this lesson students receive their test foods: rice, flour, dried apples, powdered egg white, peanuts, granola bar, freeze-dried onion, and coconut flakes. These foods were selected because they are familiar to students, they can easily be stored in the classroom for long periods of time, and they provide a wide range of test results.

LESSON 2

In addition, students receive some of the laboratory equipment they will use throughout the unit. And, they are introduced to a numbering system for organizing this equipment that will help keep their liquid and food samples and their testing materials separated. An important reason to keep these materials organized is to prevent contamination. As students conduct investigations throughout the unit, they will discover that contamination is one factor that can significantly affect test results.

In most cases, it won't be difficult for students to avoid contamination. For example, forceps have been provided so that students can handle test papers and foods without using their fingers. If some students have difficulty manipulating the forceps, you can encourage them to try to keep their fingers wiped clean.

Materials

For each student
- 1 science notebook
- 1 **Record Sheet 2-A, Test Food Observations Table**

For every two students
- 1 resealable plastic bag ("lab bag"), 20.3 cm x 25.4 cm (8" x 10")
- 1 ten-section test tray, with sections numbered 1 through 10
- 2 forceps
- 1 hand lens

For every four students
- 1 resealable plastic bag ("food bag"), 20.3 cm x 25.4 cm (8" x 10")
- 8 60 ml (2 oz) plastic cups with lids, labeled by teacher* and filled with the following foods:
    1. rice
    2. flour
    3. dried apple
    4. powdered egg white
    5. peanuts
    6. granola bar
    7. freeze-dried onion
    8. coconut flakes
- *16 labels on the food cups and lids (see Figure 2-1 and Step 4 in the **Preparation** section)
- 8 small spoons
- 1 large resealable plastic bag ("storage bag"), 30.5 cm x 38.1 cm (12" x 15"), in which to store lab bags and food bags

For the class
- 1 fine-point, permanent black marker
- Cleanup materials (2 plastic-lined disposal boxes or wastebaskets, extra paper towels, sponges)
- Soapy water (sink or buckets)
- Clear water (sink or buckets)
- Class Venn diagram from Lesson 1, "Foods We Eat for Different Meals" and large marker

LESSON 2

Figure 2-1

Test foods

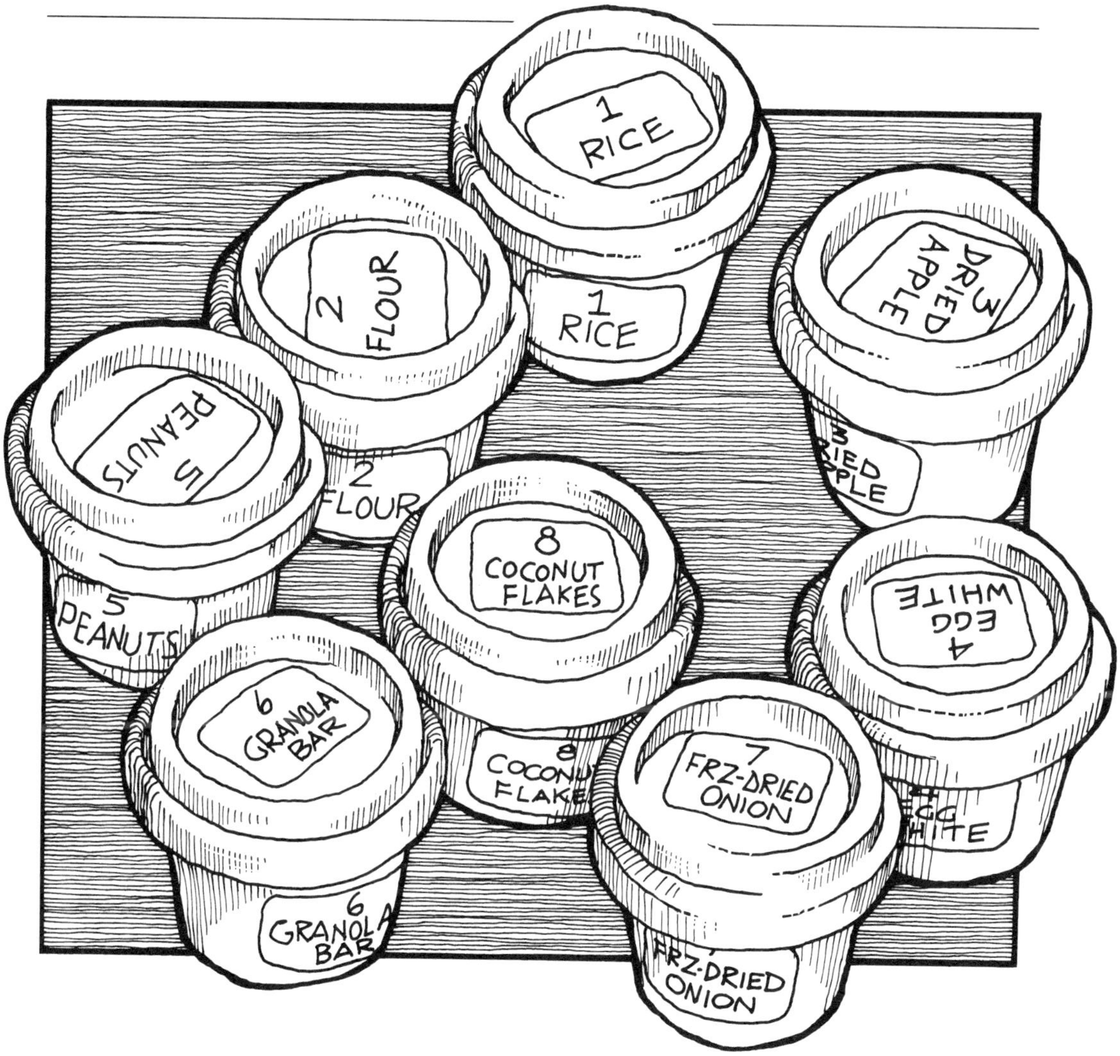

Preparation

1. Make one copy of **Record Sheet 2-A, Test Food Observations Table** for each student.
2. Using the fine-point permanent marker, number the sections in each of the ten-section test trays (see Figure 2-2).

Figure 2-2

Ten-section test tray

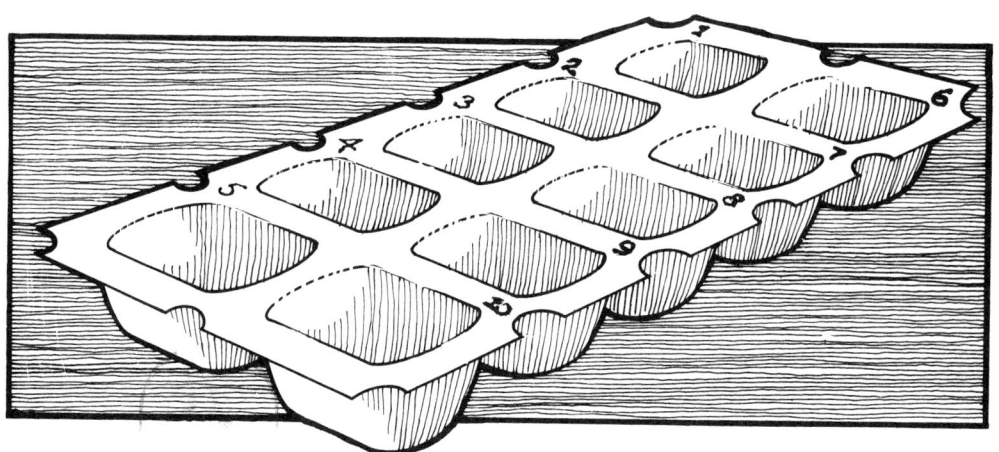

STC / *Food Chemistry*
Identifying Healthy Foods: Getting Ready / 25

LESSON 2

Figure 2-3

Distribution center for lab bags

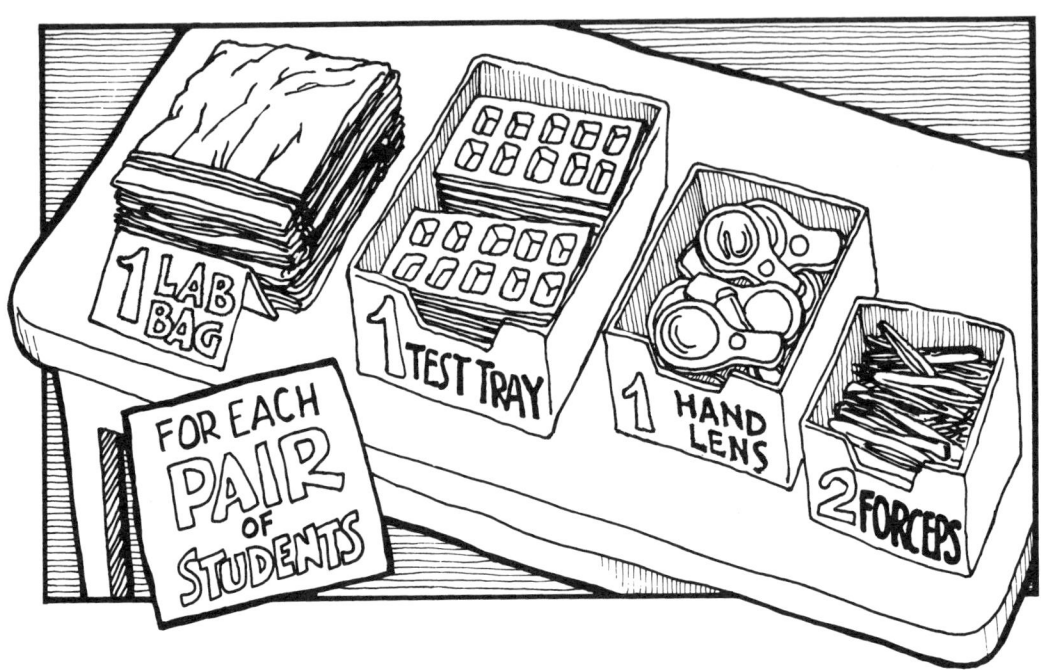

3. Set up a distribution center for the lab bags. Each pair of students will pick up one 8" x 10" resealable plastic bag (the lab bag) as well as the following materials:

   ■ 1 ten-section test tray
   ■ 1 hand lens
   ■ 2 forceps

   Arrange the materials "cafeteria style" so that students can pick up the items they need. Place a label in front of each set of materials, identifying what the material is and how many to take (see Figure 2-3).

4. Prepare the test foods using the following directions. Be sure to use either forceps or the small spoons to handle the foods, since using your fingers may affect test results.

   ■ Prepare two sets of food labels for each group of four students. Number the foods in the same sequence used in the **Materials** section:

   1. rice
   2. flour
   3. dried apple
   4. powdered egg white
   5. peanuts
   6. granola bar
   7. freeze-dried onion
   8. coconut flakes

   ■ Prepare one set (eight cups) of foods for each group of four students. Place the prepared labels on the cups and lids.

   ■ Fill each cup with the appropriate food and snap on its lid completely.

   ■ Prepare one set of eight small spoons for each group. With a fine-point permanent marker, number the handles from 1 through 8.

5. Now set up a distribution center for the test foods (see Figure 2-4). Each group of four students will pick up the following materials:
   - 1   8" x 10" resealable plastic bag (the food bag)
   - 1   set of eight foods
   - 8   small spoons
   - 1   12" x 15" resealable plastic bag in which to store the food bag and lab bags (the storage bag)

Figure 2-4

Distribution center for food bags

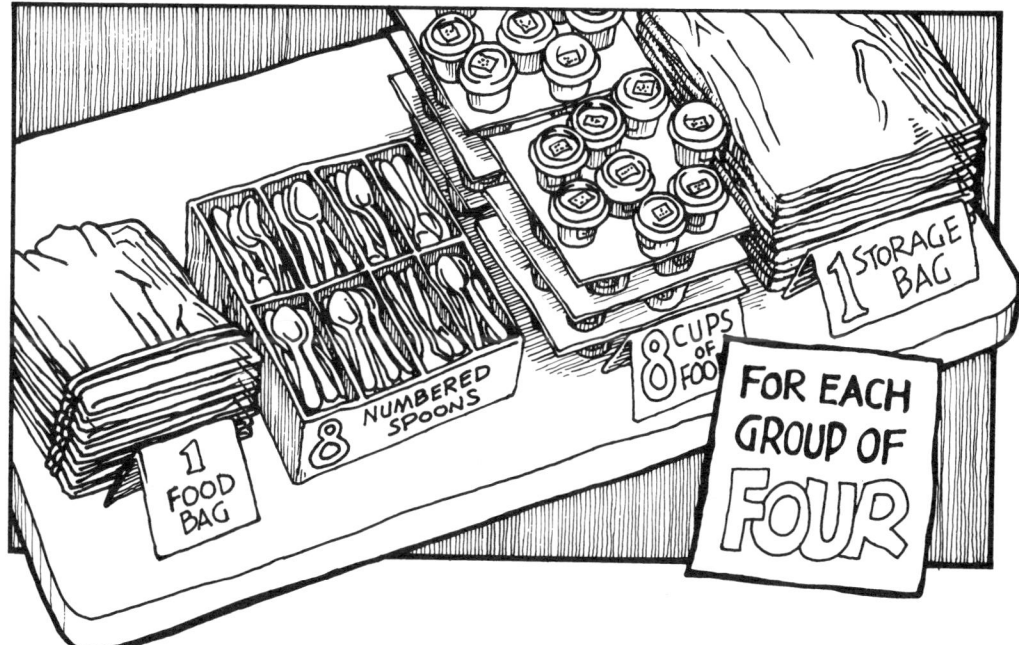

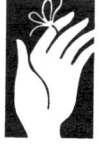

Management Tip: Students will be labeling their lab bags, food bags, and storage bags. Though only one permanent marker is called for, you may want to bring in a few extras to pass around during the labeling in this lesson and the next one, when students label their liquids bags.

6. Starting with this lesson, students will need two plastic-lined trash containers as well as other cleanup materials, such as paper towels and sponges. Have both soapy water and clear water on hand for washing and rinsing out the test trays.

7. Designate a cool, dry space for students to store the storage bags containing the lab bags and the food bags.

8. Display the class Venn diagram, "Foods We Eat for Different Meals," from Lesson 1.

LESSON 2

Procedure

1. Show the class the eight foods: rice, flour, apple, egg white, peanuts, granola bar, onion, and coconut. Then explain that over the next several weeks, the class will test these foods to discover what they contain and how their contents affect our health.

2. Next, reassemble students into their groups of four, and have them look at the class Venn diagram from Lesson 1. Ask the class which of the eight foods are on the Venn diagram at this time, and have a student add the rest.

3. Then ask the groups to discuss the following and be ready to share their ideas with the class:

   ■ From each section of the Venn diagram, select some foods you think are healthy for you. What is it about these foods that makes you think they are healthy?

   ■ What could you do to determine some of the things these foods contain that may affect your health? (Students might say "Read books," "Ask my mom," "Look at food labels," or "Do some experiments to find out what is in the foods.")

4. After groups have discussed the questions for a few minutes, have them share their ideas with the class.

5. Explain that now students will observe each of the foods by looking, feeling, smelling, and listening. Also explain that, in science, we do not use our sense of taste to make observations. Pass out **Record Sheet 2-A, Test Food Observations Table** and review it with the class. Also refer students to pg. 7 in their Student Activity Books, which shows how to use the sense of smell in science (see Figure 2-5).

Figure 2-5

Using our sense of smell in science

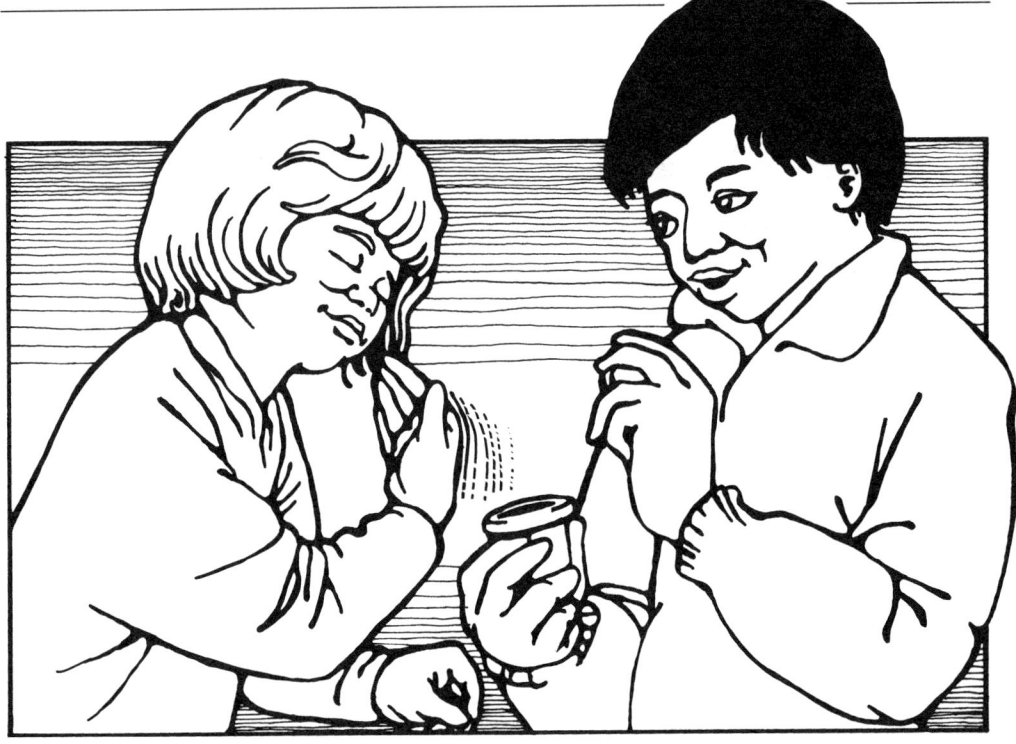

6. Before students begin their observations, they need to assemble their lab bags. Ask a student from each pair to go to the distribution center to pick up a resealable 8" x 10" plastic bag and fill it with the following:

   - 1 ten-section test tray
   - 2 pairs of forceps
   - 1 hand lens

The other student from each pair should then write "Lab Bag" and both partners' names on the label on the lab bag (see Figure 2-6). You may want to explain to the class that "lab" is short for laboratory, and briefly discuss what a laboratory is.

Figure 2-6

Labeling the lab bag

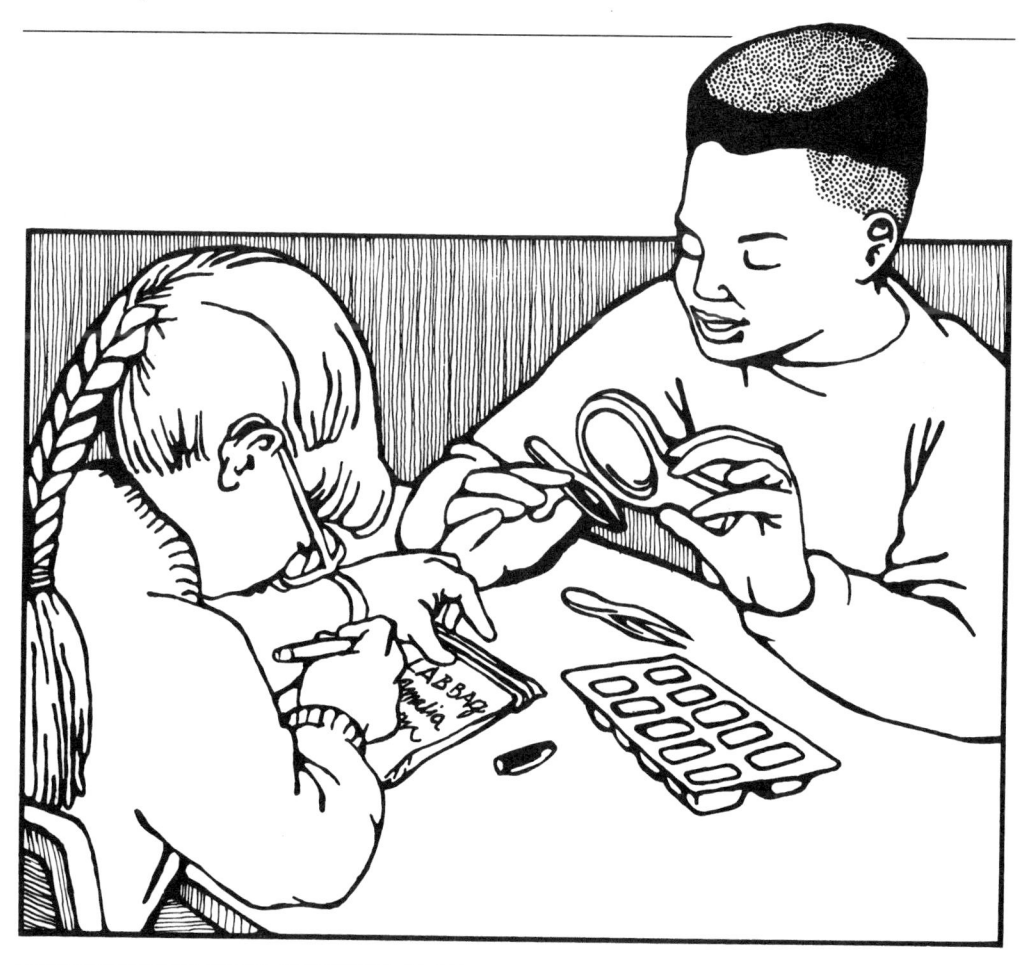

7. Now have students assemble their food bags. Ask one student from each group to pick up the following:

   - 1 8" x 10" resealable plastic bag (the food bag)
   - 1 set of the eight foods
   - 1 set of eight numbered spoons
   - 1 12" x 15" resealable plastic bag (the storage bag)

Another student should write the words "Food Bag" on the small bag containing the foods and spoons and write the group members' names on the large bag, which will be the group's storage bag throughout the unit.

LESSON 2

8. Ask each group to observe its foods. Point out the following:

   - Each of the eight food cups and lids is numbered, and so are the sections in the test tray. Foods need to be placed in tray sections that match their numbers. Let students know that they will soon discover the purpose of sections 9 and 10.

   - With each set of foods are eight small spoons, which are also numbered. For each test, be sure to match the foods with the spoons that have the same numbers.

9. Have each group discuss and agree on a way to take turns measuring out the foods. Then ask students to put a spoonful of each food in its section of the test tray to observe. Remind students always to match the numbers on the food cup, the spoon, and the tray section.

10. Allow time for students to complete **Record Sheet 2-A**. Encourage students to observe each food, first using just their eyes and then using a hand lens. Then ask several students to share their observations of each food with the class.

11. About ten minutes before the end of the class, ask students to follow these cleanup instructions:

    - Throw away the food in the test tray.
    - Wash and rinse the test tray and spoons and dry them with a paper towel.
    - Return the test tray, forceps, and hand lens to the lab bag.
    - Return the sealed food cups and spoons to the food bag.
    - Place the lab bags and the food bag in the storage bag.
    - Return the storage bag to the storage area.

Final Activities

1. Hold a class discussion about these two questions:

   - What did you learn by observing the foods? (Students may say things such as: "Powdered egg whites don't look like real eggs," "Dried apples are the most squeezable," "Rice is hard," and "The freeze-dried onions don't smell like real onions.")

   - Why is it important to number the equipment consistently for testing?

   As they discuss the equipment, some students may have trouble grasping the idea that contamination may affect test results. If so, have a couple of those students who do understand volunteer to explain or demonstrate this idea to their classmates.

2. Ask each group to choose two foods from home they would like to test and study. Make sure they decide on foods that can be stored in the classroom. Also make sure students understand who is bringing in each food. Students will begin using these foods in Lesson 4.

3. Finally, explain to students that in the next two lessons they will use the equipment they have just organized to test liquids and foods for the presence of an important nutrient—starch. Assign the students to find out as much as they can about starch before the next lesson. You may want to have them work on this during language arts time, library time, or for homework.

LESSON 2

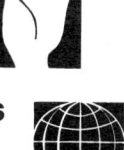

Management Tip: Lesson 3 also requires some extra advance preparation time. Again, you may want to ask a student or parent volunteer to help.

Extensions

1. Have students find out more about any one of the test foods; for example, Where does this food come from? Where is it grown? Who harvests it? How is it prepared before it is eaten? Students can write mini-reports for a class "Foods" bulletin board, or make oral presentations to the class.

2. Ask students to share what they know about other situations in which contamination can be a problem. For example, some students may have had to repeat a throat culture or urine culture because it was inadvertently exposed to other bacteria. Or, students may have read about contamination caused by nuclear meltdowns or nuclear waste.

3. Ask students to keep a record for one day of all the foods they eat for breakfast, lunch, and dinner. Then ask them to circle the ones they think are healthy. Have students date their lists and save them until the end of the unit. When they look back at their lists, will they still think the same foods are healthy?

LESSON 2

Record Sheet 2-A

Name: _____

Date: _____

Test Food Observations Table

Food	Observations	I have eaten this food before.	I have not eaten this food before.
1. Rice			
2. Flour			
3. Apple			
4. Egg White			
5. Peanut			
6. Granola Bar			
7. Onion			
8. Coconut			

STC / *Food Chemistry*

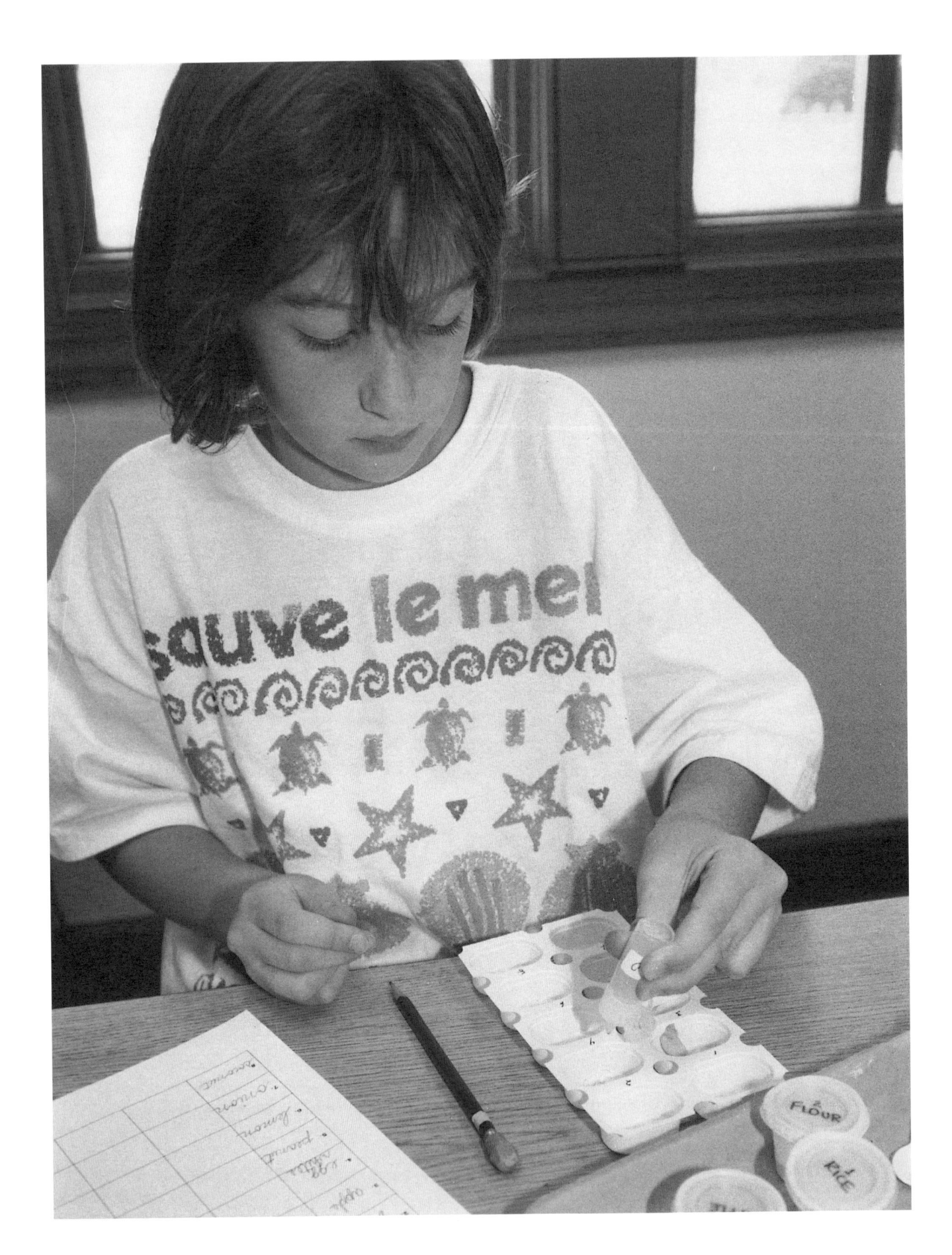

LESSON 3

Testing Liquids for Starch

Overview and Objectives

Chemical tests are used by nutritionists and others to determine the nutritional value of foods. This lesson begins a cycle of lessons in which students learn a chemical test for the nutrient starch. Specifically, students use iodine to test for the presence of starch in five liquids. In doing this, they discover how to identify a positive and negative test for starch. This will help them analyze results when they apply the same test to foods in Lesson 4. Working in teams, students get an opportunity to practice important science skills: observing, collecting and recording data, and discussing results.

- Students report on what they have discovered about starch through their individual research.

- Students make predictions, test the liquids for the presence or absence of starch, and record their results on the **Starch Test for Liquids Table**.

- Students analyze their test data to establish a positive and negative test for starch.

- Students record, analyze, and discuss the class data, identifying possible reasons for varying results.

Background

Rice, corn, and potatoes are major sources of starch, and, like most starchy foods, they also contain minerals and vitamins. Starch belongs to the category of nutrients known as carbohydrates and is made up of a long, linked chain of simple sugars. These sugars are called glucose. During digestion, our body breaks down starch into glucose, and the glucose then provides energy for our muscles and brain. Your class will study glucose in Lessons 6, 7, and 8.

Some starchy foods are also high in fiber. Fiber is indigestible material that helps move matter through the digestive tract. Fruits, vegetables, and whole grains are some sources of fiber.

In this lesson, students use iodine, a chemical that will react by changing color in the presence of starch, to establish a positive and negative test for starch. To test for starch, students will add iodine to five different liquids: cornstarch, corn syrup, corn oil, milk, and water. When they test the cornstarch, students will observe that the iodine and cornstarch mixture turns from brown to purple-black, indicating the presence of starch. This is considered a positive (+) test, and it establishes the purple-black color as the standard for determining that a food does contain starch. When students test the other liquids, however, the iodine and liquid mixture will not turn purple-black, indicating the absence of starch. This is considered a negative (−) test.

Both results give important information about the material being tested. In Lesson 4, students will test the eight foods for starch and use the results they have obtained from the liquids test to compare and interpret results. However, since the amount of starch present in foods varies, the degree of purple in a positive result will also vary. This important concept of quantifying results is addressed again in Lessons 6, 9, and 12, when students test the liquids again to establish a positive and negative test for glucose, fats, and proteins.

In each case, students will test the five liquids to identify a positive and negative test for a particular nutrient and then test foods for the presence of that nutrient. They will retest those foods for which differing results were obtained. Figure 3-1 shows the most extreme positive results possible for each nutrient. Water is included as a control and will show no change during tests for the identified nutrients.

Figure 3-1

Positive Test Table

Nutrient	Source	Test Material	Positive Test
Starch	Cornstarch	Iodine	Iodine turns from brown to purple-black in presence of starch
Glucose	Corn syrup	Glucose test paper	Test paper turns from yellow to green in presence of glucose
Fat	Corn oil	Brown paper	Corn oil leaves stain on brown paper
Protein	Milk	Coomassie blue paper (protein test paper)	Coomassie blue paper remains blue in presence of protein

Your students will be conducting many tests and recording, organizing, and interpreting many results. Record sheets (e.g., **Record Sheet 3-A, Starch Test for Liquids Table**, on pg. 49), will provide a guide to them for organizing this information, enabling them to list the liquids and their test results in the same order for each test. Figure 3-2 illustrates how a completed table will look at the end of the starch test.

As you can see, the table for this lesson also includes columns for both first test and second test results. When the class shares test results, some students may find that their results are discrepant; that is, different from the results of most others. When students retest foods for which results have been discrepant, they will record the latter results in the second test results column. By retesting, students may discover that their results were affected by careless lab procedures (e.g., mixing up spoons and causing contamination, or measuring incorrectly). In addition, during this lesson, students will become aware that the amount of a nutrient occurring in a particular food may also affect test results.

LESSON 3

Figure 3-2

Sample of a completed table

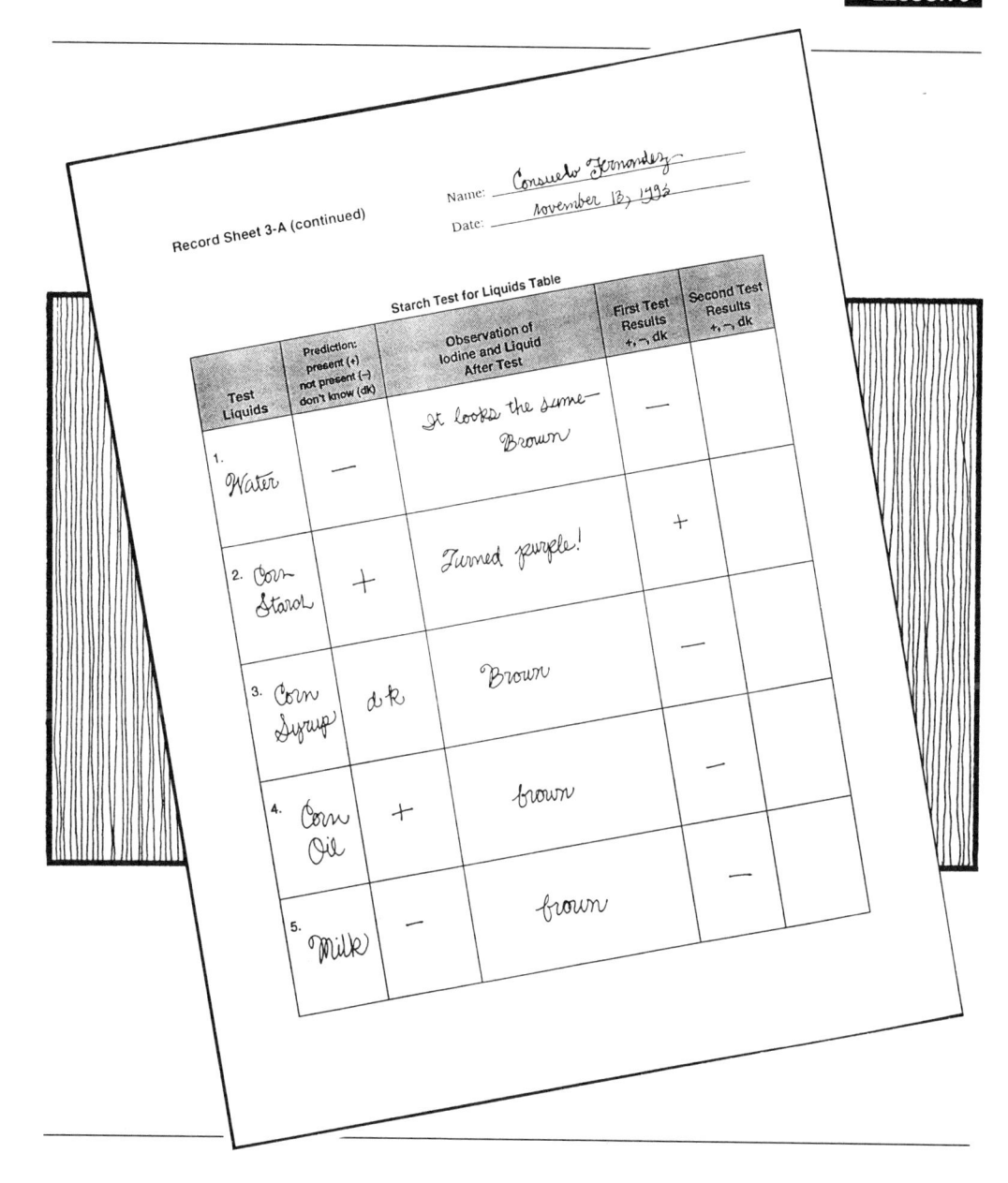

Record Sheet 3-A (continued)

Name: Consuelo Fernandez
Date: November 13, 1992

Starch Test for Liquids Table

Test Liquids	Prediction: present (+) not present (−) don't know (dk)	Observation of Iodine and Liquid After Test	First Test Results +, −, dk	Second Test Results +, −, dk
1. Water	−	It looks the same—Brown		−
2. Corn Starch	+	Turned purple!	+	
3. Corn Syrup	dk	Brown		−
4. Corn Oil	+	brown		−
5. Milk	−	brown		

Note: In Lesson 5, the class will read the first of several **Reading Selections** that explain how the different nutrients affect health and nutrition. For more in-depth information about starch at this time, you may want to take a look at the **Reading Selection** on pg. 65. The references listed in the **Bibliography** in **Appendix B** may also be helpful.

Materials

For each student
  1 science notebook
  1 **Record Sheet 3-A, Starch Test for Liquids**

For every four students
  1 storage bag containing the following:
      2 lab bags
      1 food bag

LESSON 3

1 resealable plastic bag ("liquids bag"), 20.3 cm × 25.4 cm (8 × 10")
2 six-section test trays, with sections numbered 1 through 5
5 dropper bottles, labeled by teacher* and filled with the following test liquids:
   1. water
   2. cornstarch
   3. corn syrup
   4. corn oil
   5. milk
*6 labels on dropper bottles (see Step 3 in the **Preparation** section)
1 labeled dropper bottle of dilute iodine
1 box of toothpicks

For the class

1 carton of skim milk, 237 ml (½ pt)
1 bottle of tincture of iodine, 30 ml (1 oz)
1 amber bottle, 250 ml (½ pt)
1 graduated plastic dropper
5 funnels
2 clean jars with lids, for mixing 100 ml (3½ oz) quantities of liquid cornstarch and dilute corn syrup
1 measuring spoon, 5 ml (1 tsp)
1 graduated plastic cup, 100 ml (4½ oz)
1 sheet of newsprint or poster board (for "Class Liquids Test Table") and large marker
1 fine-point permanent marker
  Newsprint or poster board, or an overhead transparency and pen (see Step 1 in the **Procedure** section)
  Cleanup materials (2 plastic-lined disposal boxes, paper towels, sponges)
  Soapy water (sink or buckets)
  Clear water (sink or buckets)

Preparation

1. Make one copy of **Record Sheet 3-A, Starch Test for Liquids** for each student.

2. On a large sheet of newsprint make a table entitled "Class Liquids Test Table" (see Figure 3-3).

3. Prepare and apply a set of six dropper bottle labels—one for each liquid—for each group of four students. Number and label the test liquids as follows: 1. water, 2. cornstarch, 3. corn syrup, 4. corn oil, 5. milk. Do not number the iodine labels.

4. Mix your iodine test solution as follows:

   ■ Fill the amber bottle to the shoulder with water.

   ■ Using the dropper, add 10 ml of tincture of iodine.

   ■ Cap the bottle and shake it gently to mix the solution.

   Test the solution on a little cornstarch to be sure it produces the purple-black color that makes iodine an effective indicator.

5. Using one of the funnels, fill all of the iodine dropper bottles from the 0.1% iodine solution stored in the amber bottle (see Figure 3-4).

Figure 3-3

CLASS LIQUIDS TEST TABLE

TEST LIQUIDS	RESULTS OF STARCH TEST	RESULTS OF GLUCOSE TEST	RESULTS OF FATS TEST	RESULTS OF PROTEINS TEST
WATER				
CORN STARCH				
CORN SYRUP				
CORN OIL				
MILK				

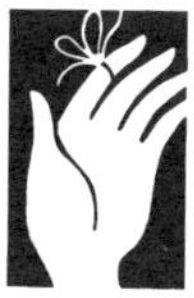

Management Tip: You will use the iodine solution again in Lessons 4, 5, and 16. Keep in mind, however, that iodine solution is sensitive to air and light, so it may lose its potency after being in the small dropper bottles for a few weeks. Before each use, test the iodine solution on a small amount of cornstarch. If no color change occurs, pour the iodine in the dropper bottle down the drain and add fresh solution from the amber bottle. Because the iodine is a natural substance and a very weak solution, discarding it in this way is acceptable.

Note: You can usually remove iodine stains from clothing by rubbing the material with lemon juice or with vitamin C tablets dissolved in water.

6. Prepare the cornstarch and the corn syrup according to the following directions.

   - Cornstarch: Mix together 5 ml (1 tsp) of cornstarch and 100 ml (3½ oz) of tap water.
   - Corn syrup: Mix together 5 ml (1 tsp) of corn syrup and 100 ml (3½ oz) of tap water.

7. Obtain 237 ml (½ pint) of skim milk.

LESSON 3

Figure 3-4

Using the funnel

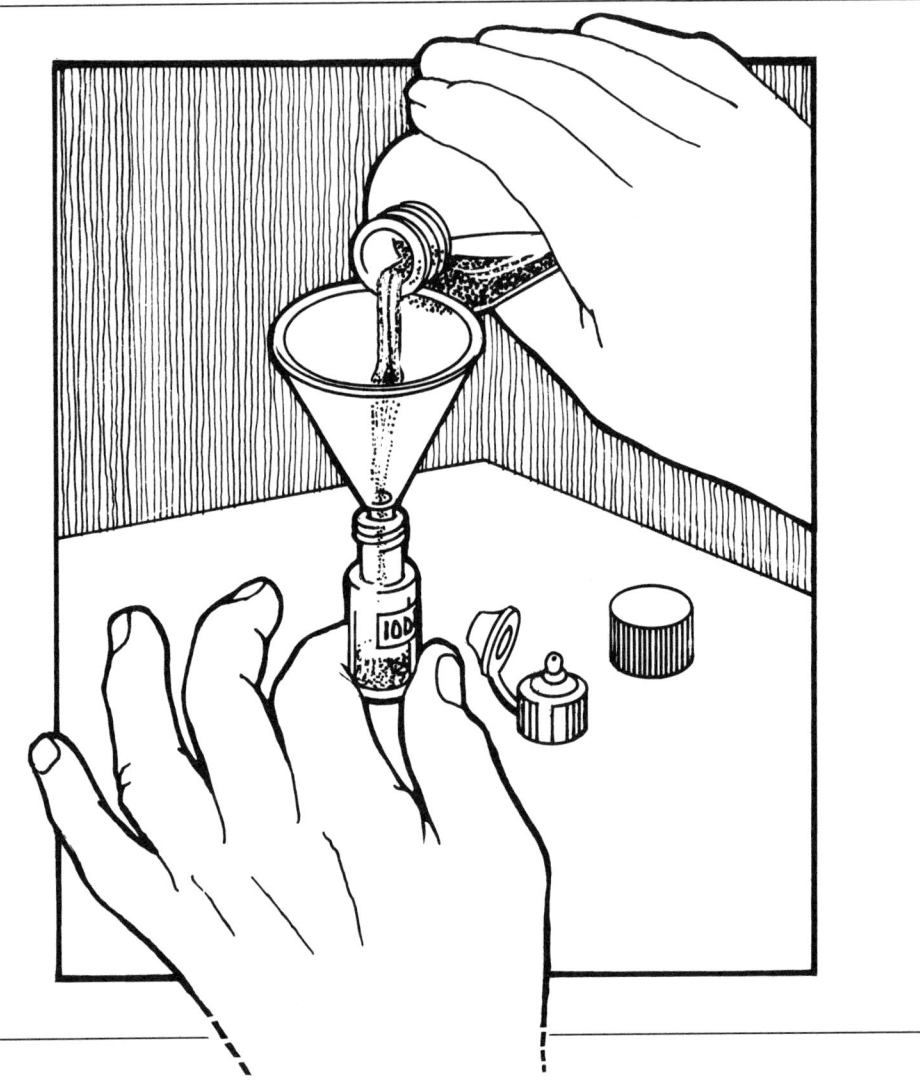

8. Using a different funnel for each liquid (except water), fill the appropriate dropper bottles with the appropriate liquids (water, cornstarch, corn syrup, corn oil, and milk) and make sure to fasten the caps securely.

9. Using the fine-point permanent marker, number five of the sections in the six-section test tray (see Figure 3-5).

10. Set up a distribution center for the liquids bags (see Figure 3-6). One student from each group of **four** should pick up the following materials:

   - 1   storage bag from Lesson 2, containing the lab bags and the food bag

   - 1   8" × 10" resealable plastic bag ("liquids bag"), in which to put the following:

      2   six-section test trays

      1   set of five test liquids

      1   dropper bottle of iodine

      1   box of toothpicks

11. If you do not have access to a sink, prepare several buckets of soapy water and clear water in which students can wash and rinse out their test trays at the end of the period.

LESSON 3

Figure 3-5

Six-section test tray

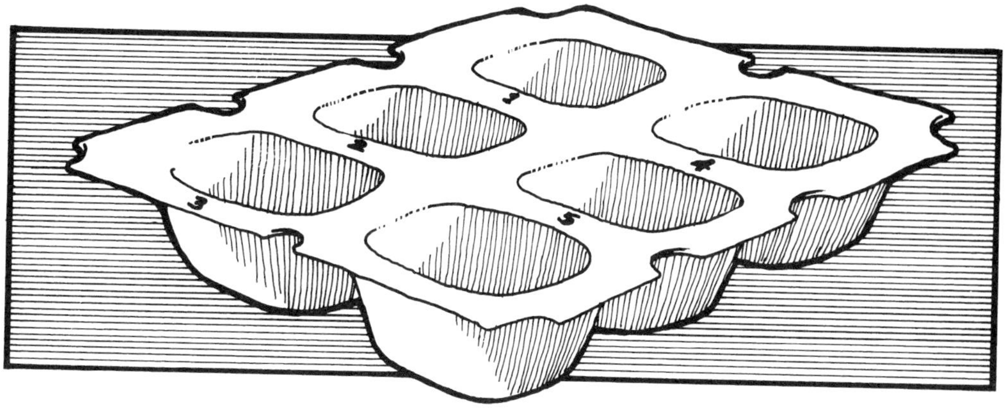

Procedure

1. Begin this lesson by asking students to share what they found out about starch. Record students' ideas on newsprint or an overhead transparency. Or, ask students quickly to record a few ideas in their notebooks.

2. Then briefly explain that students will test five liquids with iodine to identify a positive and negative test for starch. And they will use this data when testing their foods for starch in Lesson 4. Show the class one of the bottles of iodine, and explain that when the iodine is mixed with a material that contains starch, a chemical reaction will occur. In this case, the iodine and liquid mixture will change color from brown to purple-black.

   Note: Some of your students may not understand the concept of positive (+) and negative (–) tests. Take a few minutes to talk with the class about what both terms mean.

3. Following this introduction, hand out **Record Sheet 3-A, Starch Test for Liquids**. Review the purpose of the table with the class, discussing what data should be written in each column. Tell the class to use only the "first test" column for now.

Figure 3-6

Distribution center for liquids bags

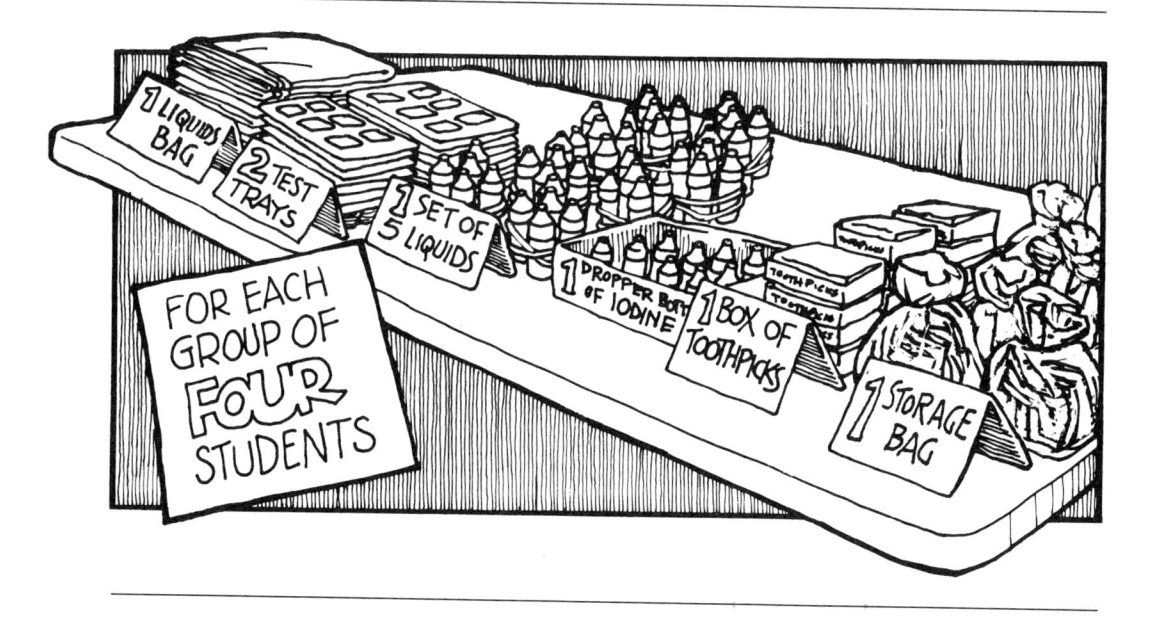

STC / *Food Chemistry*

Testing Liquids for Starch / **41**

LESSON 3

Note: When you review test instructions with the class, you will note that the children are told to put a drop of iodine into the unnumbered section of the test tray. This serves as the **control**, an unchanged basis for comparison. Students will compare the control and the chemical changes they observe.

4. Next, review the **Student Instructions for Testing the Liquids for Starch** (on pg. 46 of this guide and on pg. 12 of the Student Activity Book).

5. Now, have one student from each group of four go to the distribution center to pick up a resealable 8" x 10" plastic bag and fill it with the following items (see Figure 3-7):

   - 1 dropper bottle of each test liquid: water, cornstarch, corn syrup, corn oil, and milk
   - 1 dropper bottle of iodine
   - 2 six-section test trays
   - 1 box of toothpicks

   Also have the student pick up his or her group's storage bag. Ask another student to write "Liquids Bag" on the small bag. Then let students get to work.

Figure 3-7

Filling the liquids bag

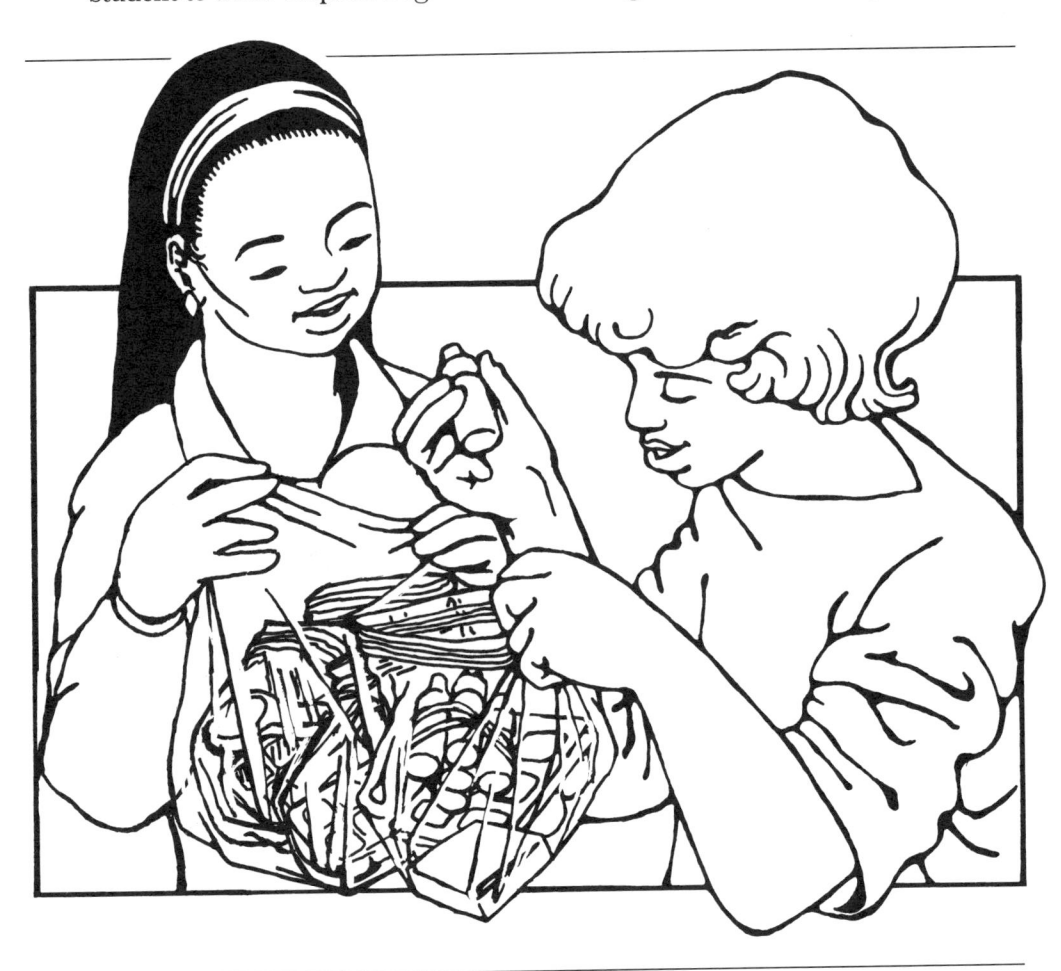

42 / Testing Liquids for Starch

STC / *Food Chemistry*

LESSON 3

6. After completing their investigations and recording results, students need to follow these cleanup directions (also on pg. 10 of the Student Activity Book):

    - Throw away used toothpicks.
    - Empty and rinse out the dropper bottles of cornstarch, corn syrup, and milk.
    - Wipe the test trays with paper towels, rinse them out, and then wipe them again.
    - Place the dropper bottles, test trays, and box of toothpicks in the liquids bag. Place the liquids bag in your team's storage bag and return it to the storage area.

Figure 3-8

Adding results to the "Class Liquids Test Table"

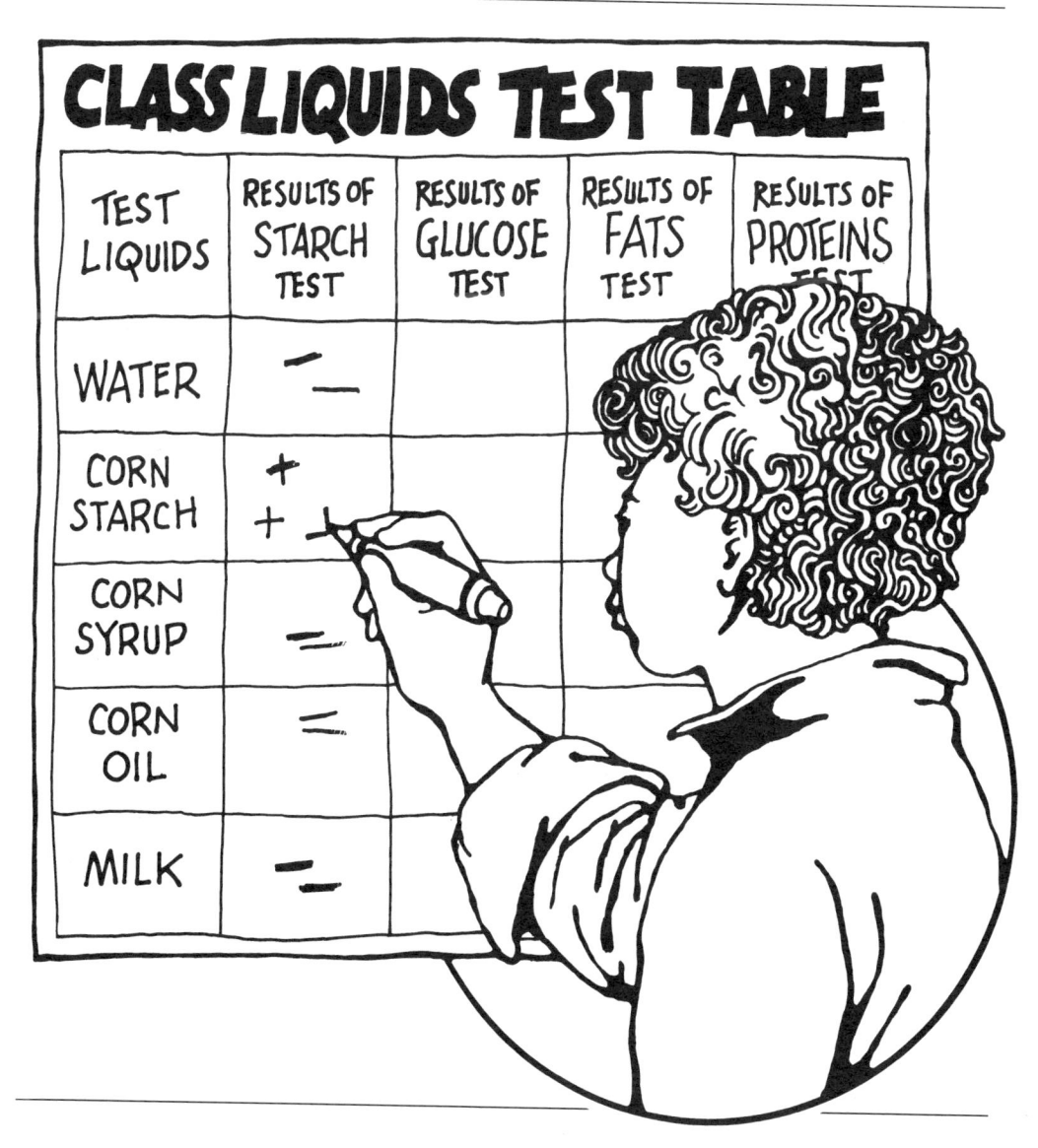

CLASS LIQUIDS TEST TABLE

TEST LIQUIDS	RESULTS OF STARCH TEST	RESULTS OF GLUCOSE TEST	RESULTS OF FATS TEST	RESULTS OF PROTEINS TEST
WATER	−			
CORN STARCH	+ +			
CORN SYRUP	−			
CORN OIL	−			
MILK	−			

Final Activities

1. Now introduce the purpose of the "Class Liquids Test Table." Ask one member from each group to record his or her group's results (+ or −) in the starch column (see Figure 3-8).

2. Then, starting with water, ask students to describe in detail what happened to each liquid after they added the iodine.

LESSON 3

3. Some groups' results may differ from others'. If so, ask students to talk about why they think this happened. If there are discrepant results, provide time for students to repeat the test to see if they get the same results. Point out the column on their **Record Sheet** for recording second test results and explain that scientists routinely repeat their experiments to confirm that results are valid.

4. Based on the class's test results, ask which liquids contain starch and which do not. Then ask students to talk about how testing with the iodine helped them to identify which liquids contain starch. Explain that the purple-black color is the "standard" for determining the positive test for starch.

5. Ask students to write in their notebooks how testing the liquids will help them determine which foods contain starch.

6. Remind students to bring in two extra foods to test in the next lesson.

   Note: Keep the "Class Liquids Test Table." You will use it again in Lessons 6, 9, and 12.

Extensions

1. Have students find out if the color change indicating a positive test for starch depends on the amount of starch present. Do the following test.
   - To sections one through four in the six-section test tray, add, respectively, one, two, three, and four drops of liquid cornstarch.
   - To these same sections, in the same order, add three, two, one, and zero drops of water.
   - Then add two drops of iodine to each section.
   - Record and present your findings.

2. Have students conduct research about iodine, finding out where it comes from and what other uses it has (such as why it is often added to salt).

3. Invite students to bring in recipes that contain starchy foods. Compile these into a starch cookbook.

Assessments

This lesson is the beginning of the cycle in which students test for different nutrients, first by testing the liquids to establish what constitutes a positive result, and then by testing the foods. Over the coming lessons, watch for student growth in the following areas.

Lab Procedures
- Do students avoid contamination by matching the numbers on the different test materials?
- Do students avoid contamination by using a new toothpick to stir each liquid or food?
- Do students set up a control and use it to compare and interpret results?
- Do students share materials and work together as a team?

LESSON 3

Written Work

Notebook Entries

- Using their test results, can students identify a positive starch test and a negative starch test?

- Have students described their observations of their test results?

Data Tables

- Do students know how to record test results using + and –?

- Do students understand that a positive starch test means the liquid or food contains starch and a negative test means that it doesn't?

- Can students explain how testing the liquids will help them determine which foods do and do not contain starch?

Discussions

- Do students accurately communicate the results of their investigations, both in class discussions and in written form in their notebooks?

- Do students bring up the idea of contamination?

Management Tip: Make sure that groups have brought their two foods from home in time for you to prepare them for Lesson 4.

LESSON 3

Student Instructions for Testing Liquids for Starch

1. Answer pre-lab questions 1 and 2 on **Record Sheet 3-A**.

2. Put a drop of iodine in the unnumbered section of the test tray. This is your control.

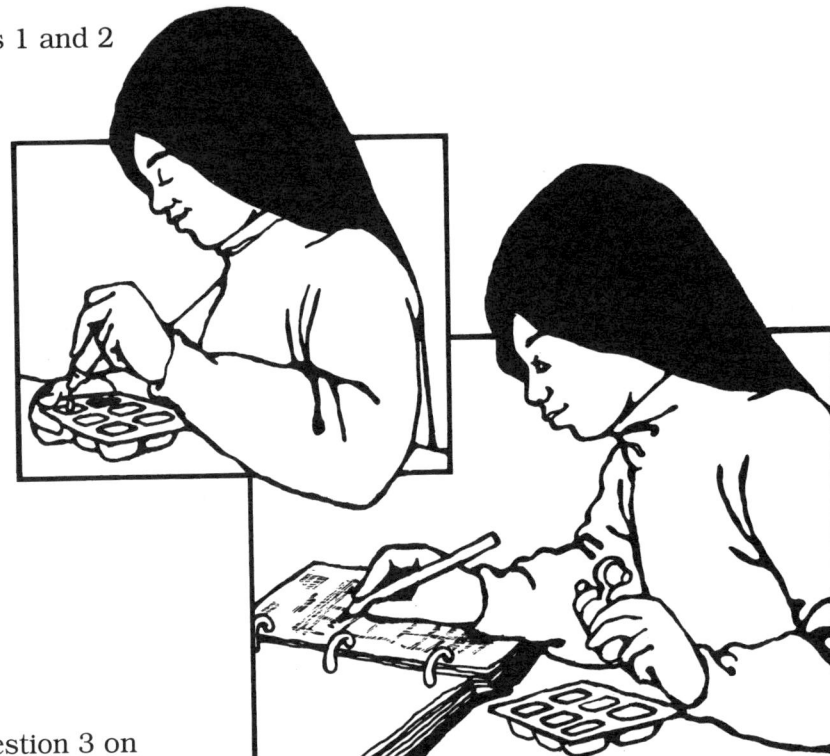

3. Then answer pre-lab question 3 on **Record Sheet 3-A**.

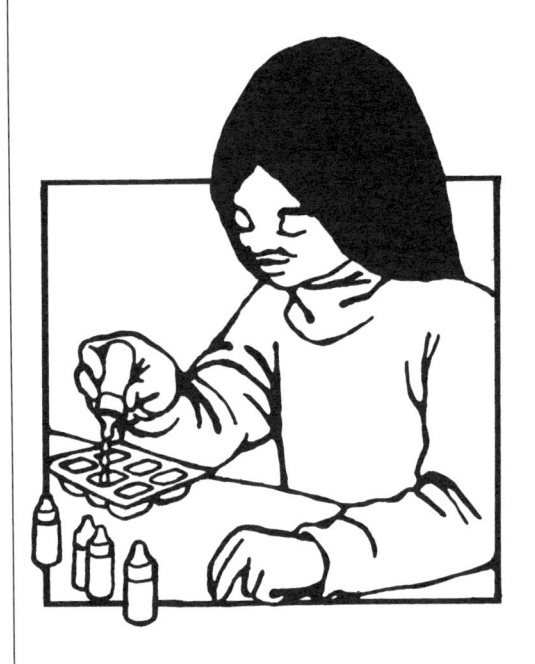

4. Put three drops of each liquid—water, cornstarch, corn syrup, corn oil, and milk—in its appropriate section of the test tray. Make sure the number of the liquid in the tray section matches the liquid's number on **Record Sheet 3-A**.

46 / Testing Liquids for Starch

STC / *Food Chemistry*

LESSON 3

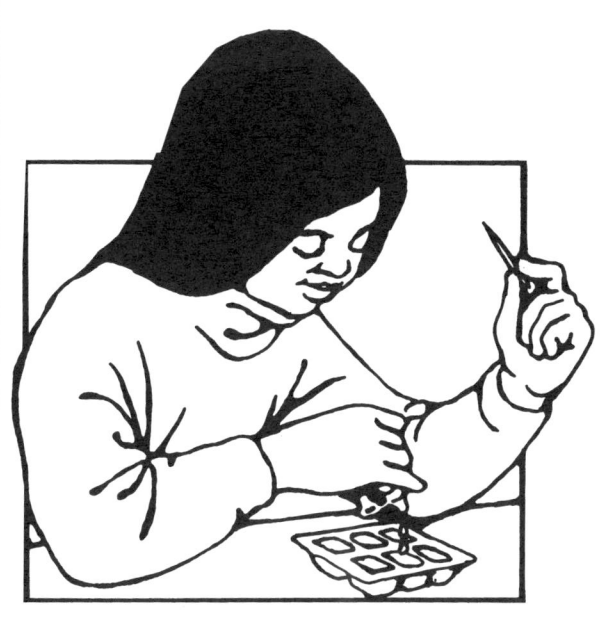

5. Put two drops of iodine into the first liquid (water) and stir the iodine and water with a toothpick.

6. After you mix the iodine and water, observe the color. Share observations with your teammates.

7. Record your observations on **Record Sheet 3-A**.

8. Then add iodine to the next liquid (cornstarch), stir with a different toothpick, and record your observations.

9. Repeat this process for the corn syrup, corn oil, and milk. Be sure to use a different toothpick for each liquid.

10. Complete the two post-lab questions.

11. Follow your cleanup instructions.

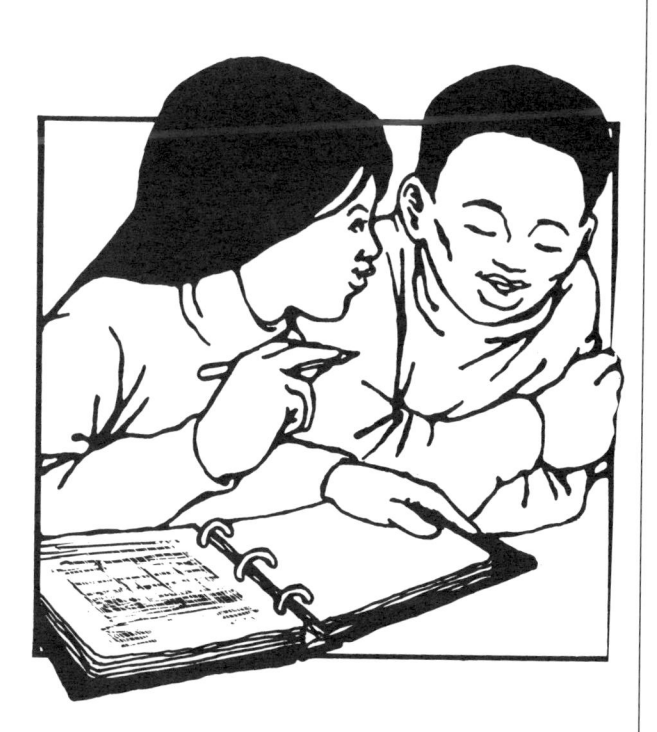

STC / *Food Chemistry*   Testing Liquids for Starch / **47**

LESSON 3

Record Sheet 3-A   Name: _____

                              Date: _____

Starch Test for Liquids

Pre-Lab Questions

1. What is the nutrient you are testing for? _____
   _____

2. What test material are you using to identify the nutrient? _____
   _____

3. What is the color of the test material before it is used? _____
   _____

Lab

Now test each liquid for starch. As you complete each test, record your results on the table on the next page. When the table is completed, answer the questions below.

Post-Lab Questions

Using your results, how can you identify a positive test (+) for starch?
_____
_____
_____

Using your results, how can you identify a negative test (–) for starch?
_____
_____
_____

STC / *Food Chemistry*

Record Sheet 3-A (continued)

Name: _____

Date: _____

Starch Test for Liquids Table

Test Liquids	Prediction: present (+) not present (−) don't know (dk)	Observation of Iodine and Liquid after Test	First Test Results +, −, dk	Second Test Results +, −, dk
1. Water				
2. Cornstarch				
3. Corn syrup				
4. Corn oil				
5. Milk				

STC / *Food Chemistry*

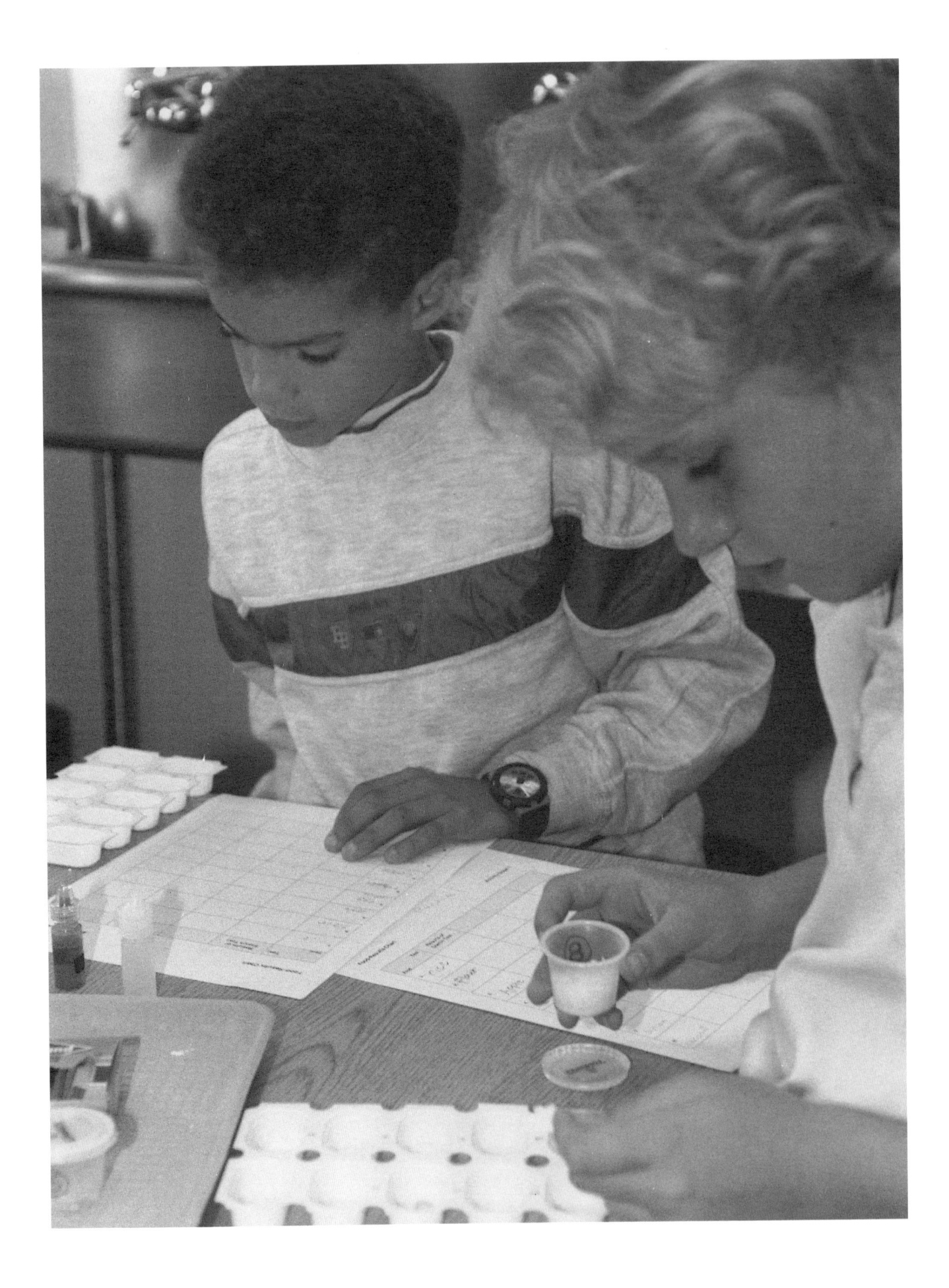

LESSON 4

Testing Foods for Starch

Overview and Objectives

In Lesson 3, students discovered that the chemical iodine can be used to identify the presence of starch in foods because iodine turns varying shades of purple-black in relation to the amount of starch in a substance. Now students will apply what they have observed to test their eight foods as well as the two additional foods they have brought from home. This activity paves the way for a discussion in Lesson 5 on why test results in the class may vary.

- Students predict which of their foods contain starch and then test the foods to see if their predictions are correct.

- Students record and organize test data on both individual Record Sheets and a class "Foods Test Table."

- In their notebooks, students record discoveries and questions about starch.

Background

In this lesson, students will receive **Record Sheet 4-A, Starch Test for Foods** on which they will organize the data their food tests generate. Figure 4-1 shows how a completed table will look at the end of this starch test.

As the data in Figure 4-1 indicate, foods such as rice and flour contain large quantities of starch and, therefore, turn purple-black when iodine is added. On the other hand, certain vegetables and fruits (such as the dried apples) contain little starch and may turn only a very faint purple-black, which then fades. These fruits and vegetables also contain vitamin C, which has a chemical reaction to iodine and causes the color to fade. Using more iodine restores the purple-black color to the apple, but not to the onion, which contains even less starch.

Materials

For each student
   1 science notebook
   1 **Record Sheet 4-A, Starch Test for Foods**

For every four students
   1 storage bag containing the following:
       2 lab bags
       1 food bag
       1 liquids bag

LESSON 4

Figure 4-1

Sample of a completed table

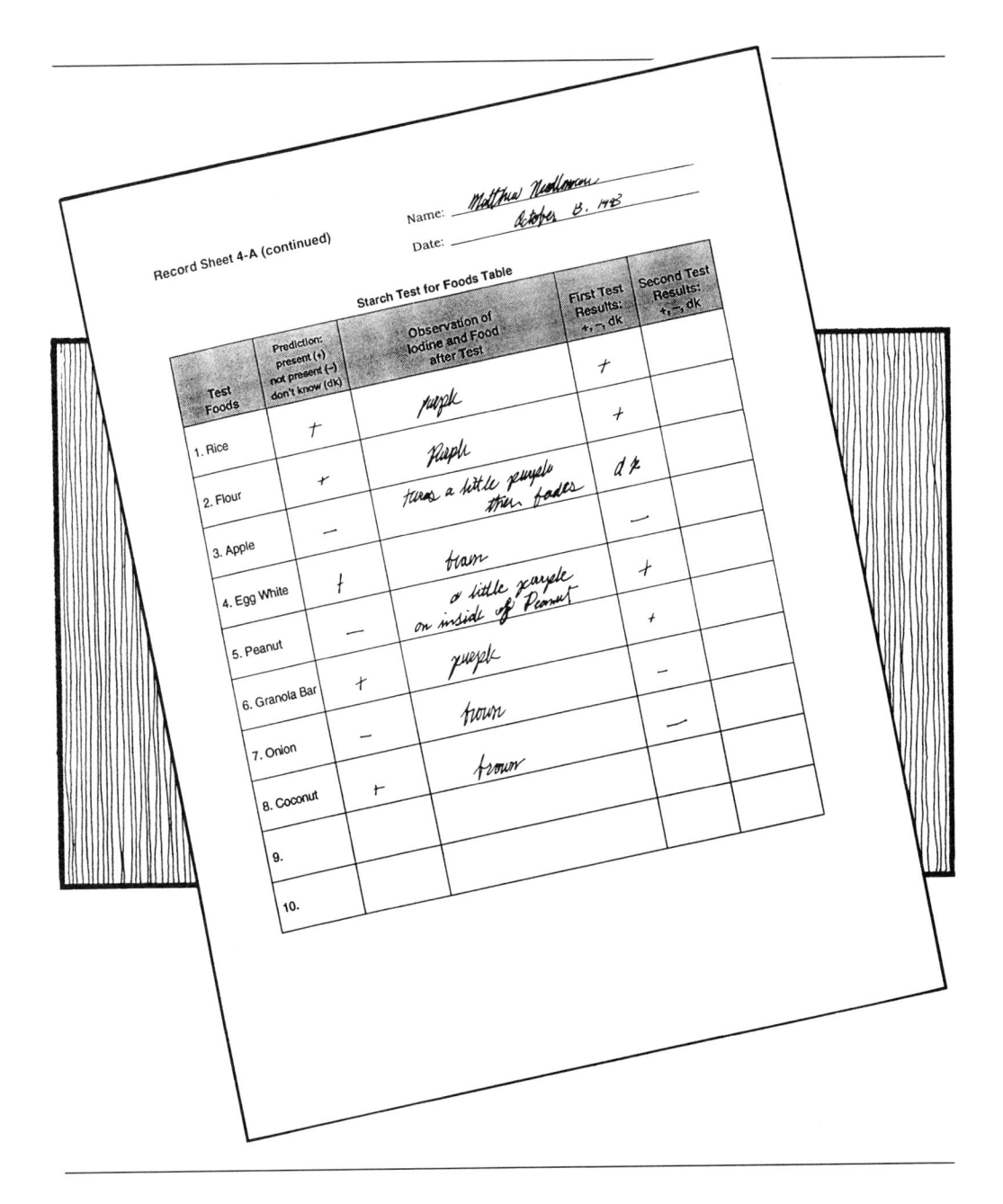

Test Foods	Prediction: present (+) not present (−) don't know (dk)	Observation of Iodine and Food after Test	First Test Results: +, −, dk	Second Test Results: +, −, dk
1. Rice	+	purple	+	
2. Flour	+	purple	+	
3. Apple	−	turns a little purple then fades	dk	
4. Egg White	+	brown	−	
5. Peanut	−	a little purple on inside of Peanut	+	
6. Granola Bar	+	purple	+	
7. Onion	−	brown	−	
8. Coconut	+	brown		
9.				
10.				

Name: Matthew ___
Date: October 8, 1993
Record Sheet 4-A (continued)
Starch Test for Foods Table

  2 plastic food cups with lids, labeled by teacher* and filled with the two foods supplied by the group
  2 small spoons (for the two foods brought from home)
  4 paper towels
 *4 labels on the new food cups and lids (see Step 3 in the **Preparation** section)

For the class

  1 sheet of newsprint or poster board (for "Class Foods Test Table") and large marker
     Cleanup materials (2 plastic-lined disposal boxes, sponge, brush, dustpan, paper towels)
     Soapy water (sink or buckets)
     Clear water (sink or buckets)

Figure 4-2

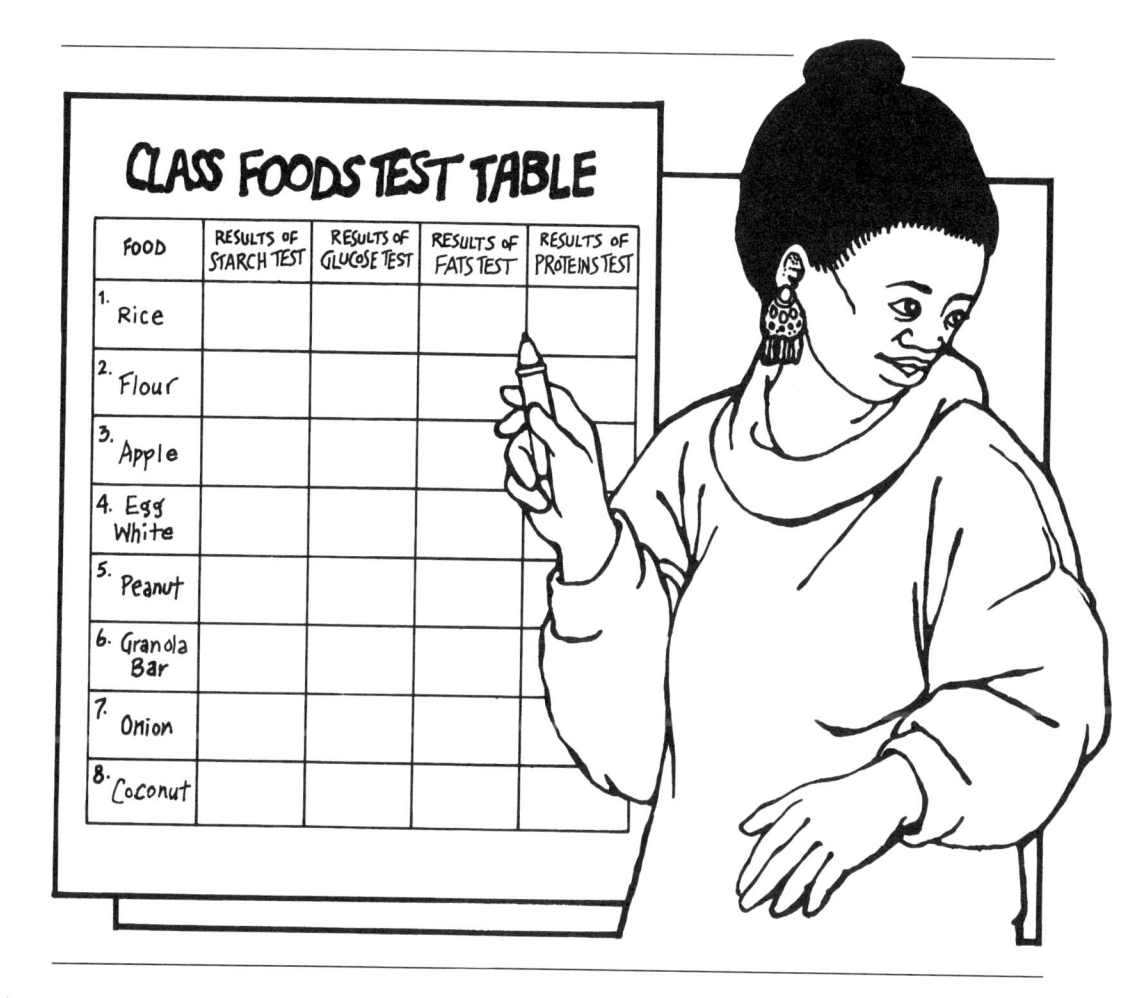

FOOD	RESULTS OF STARCH TEST	RESULTS OF GLUCOSE TEST	RESULTS OF FATS TEST	RESULTS OF PROTEINS TEST
1. Rice				
2. Flour				
3. Apple				
4. Egg White				
5. Peanut				
6. Granola Bar				
7. Onion				
8. Coconut				

CLASS FOODS TEST TABLE

Preparation

1. On a large sheet of newsprint, make the "Class Foods Test Table" (see Figure 4-2) and hang it in the classroom.

2. Make one copy of **Record Sheet 4-A, Starch Test for Foods** for each student.

3. Prepare cups with lids for foods students brought from home. Write the names of a group's new foods on labels for cups and lids. Number the foods 9 and 10, and also number each group's new spoons 9 and 10.

4. If you do not have access to a sink, prepare several buckets of soapy water and several buckets of clear water in which students can wash and then rinse out their test trays.

Procedure

1. Hold a class discussion about the following questions:

    ■ What is the procedure for testing liquids for starch?

    ■ What is the difference between a positive and negative test for starch?

    ■ What else have you learned about starch?

2. Following this review, distribute **Record Sheet 4-A, Starch Test for Foods** and briefly discuss the pre- and post-lab questions, as well as what goes in each column of the table.

LESSON 4

3. Next, have students predict if starch is present or not in each food. Remind them that a prediction is not a test and there is no right or wrong answer. Also remind students to write "don't know" (dk) if they have no prediction. Then have them record their individual predictions (+, –, or dk) in the appropriate column of the table.

4. Review the **Student Instructions for Testing Foods for Starch** on pg. 56 (also found on pg. 18 of the Student Activity Book).

Management Tips: Three foods—dried apple, peanut, and granola bars—require special preparation for testing. To peel and crumble the peanut, tear the apple, and crumble the granola bar, ask a pair of students to work together on each of the three foods. The best way to crumble a peanut without pieces flying everywhere is to hold it against the bottom of a tray section with one forceps and jab it with the clamped tip of the other forceps.

Make sure to tell students to wipe the forceps carefully with a paper towel after preparing each of these foods to avoid contamination.

5. Then, have a member from each group pick up the following materials:
   - 1 storage bag
   - 2 new cups with foods from home
   - 2 small spoons

   Let students begin their investigations.

6. When students have finished testing and recording their results, they need to clean up. Go over the following cleanup instructions (also on pg. 16 of the Student Activity Book).
   - Discard the contents of the test trays and the used toothpicks into the plastic-lined disposal boxes.
   - Put the correct lids securely on the ten cups of food.
   - Wipe the spoons with a paper towel, and return the food cups and spoons to the food bag.
   - Return the box of toothpicks and the bottles of iodine and water to the liquids bag.
   - Wash the test trays in soapy water, rinse them, and wipe them dry. Place the ten-section trays in the lab bag and the six-section trays in the liquids bag.
   - Wash, rinse, and dry the forceps and return them to the lab bag.
   - Put the lab bag, food bag, and liquids bag back in the storage bag.
   - Return the materials to the storage area.

Final Activities

1. After the cleanup, ask one student from each group to record that group's starch test results on the "Class Foods Test Table." Let students know they will discuss these results in the next lesson.

2. Then ask students to answer the following questions in their notebooks:
   - What did you discover during this investigation?
   - What surprised you?
   - What questions do you have about starch?

Extensions

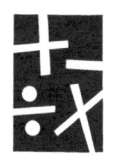

1. Have students compute and graph the cost per serving for various types of starchy foods, such as rice, beans, and pasta.

2. Explain to students that one way to remove iodine stains from clothing is to treat the material with lemon juice or vitamin C tablets dissolved in water. Challenge them to try removing iodine from a scrap of fabric. Have them share the procedure and the results with the class.

3. Ask students to talk to their parents about the foods they eat every day that contain starch and to make a list to share with the class. Suggest that they test some of these foods.

4. Have the class make starch collages using pasta, rice, and beans.

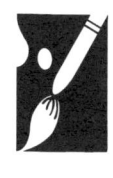

LESSON 4

Student Instructions for Testing Foods for Starch

1. Answer pre-lab questions 1 and 2 on **Record Sheet 4-A**.

2. Remove the following test materials from the storage bag.
   - Two lab bags, each containing a ten-section test tray, one hand lens, and two forceps
   - One food bag containing eight food cups and eight small spoons
   - One liquids bag containing five dropper bottles of test liquids, one dropper bottle of iodine, one box of toothpicks, and two six-section test trays

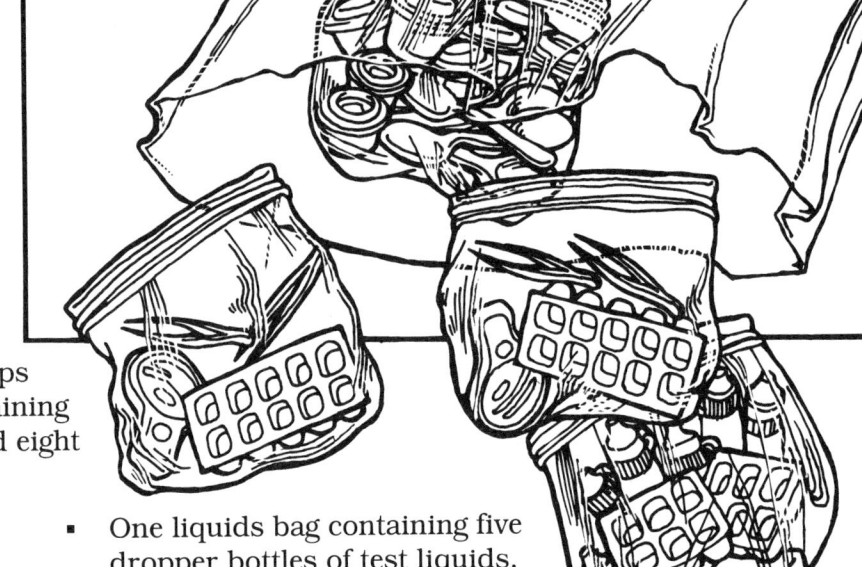

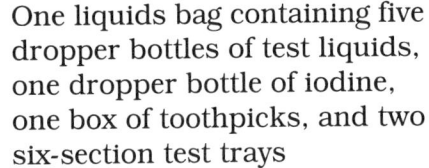

3. If your dropper bottle of water is nearly empty, add some to it.

4. Put two drops of iodine in the unnumbered section in the six-section test tray. This is your control. Observe the iodine by itself, and answer pre-lab question 3 on **Record Sheet 4-A**.

5. Some foods need preparation before testing. You and your partner may use your fingers to shell the peanut since you will not be touching the actual food. (Touching the test food with your fingers may contaminate the foods.) Use your forceps to place a shelled peanut or two and small portions of dried apple and granola into their matching numbered sections of the test tray. Then, also with forceps, do the following:
   - Tear the apple into small pieces.
   - Remove the peanut's papery skin. Hold down the peanut with forceps and have your partner use the other forceps to crumble the kernel.
   - Crumble a small piece of the granola bar.

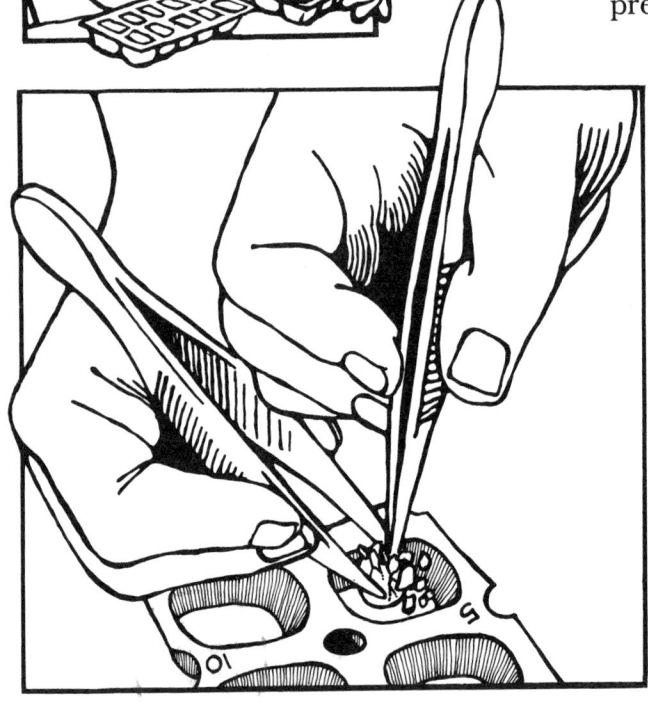

56 / Testing Foods for Starch

STC / *Food Chemistry*

LESSON 4

6. Now place one spoonful of each of the other foods into your test tray. To keep foods from mixing together, make sure the number of each spoon matches the number of the food and the test tray section you place it in.

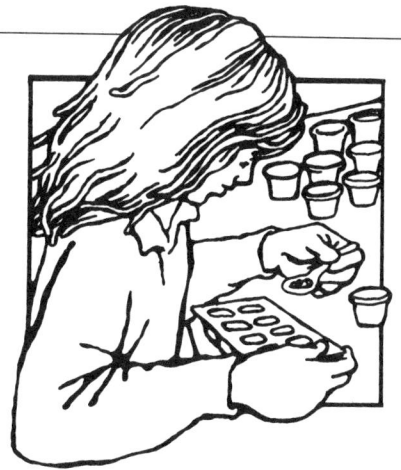

7. Now write the names of your two new test foods in the first column of your table.

8. Add two drops of water to the food in section 1 of the tray (rice).

9. Stir the rice and water well with a toothpick.

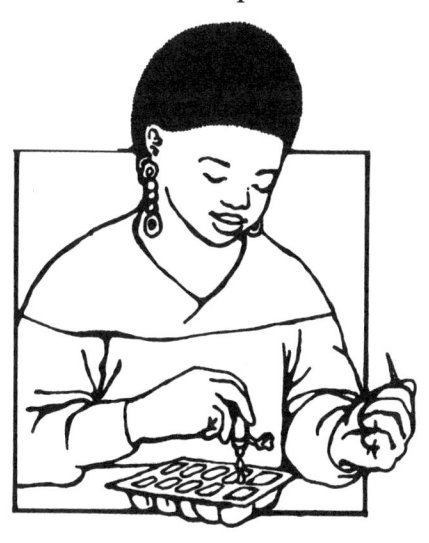

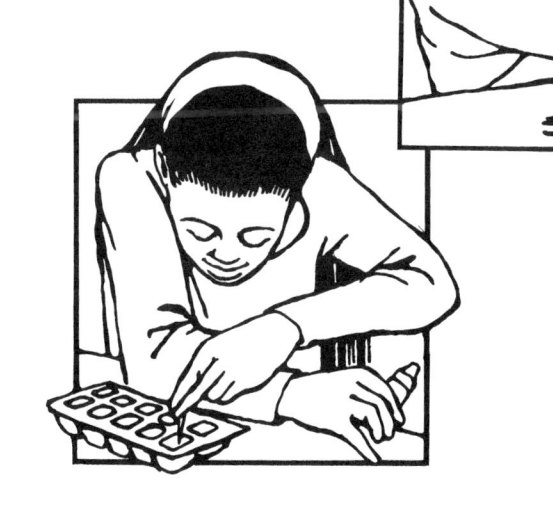

10. Repeat steps 8 and 9 with the other nine foods. (Be sure to use a different toothpick for each food.)

11. Add two drops of iodine to the rice and water. Record your observations and the test result on **Record Sheet 4-A**.

12. Repeat step 11 with the other foods.

13. Complete the post-lab questions.

14. Now follow your cleanup instructions.

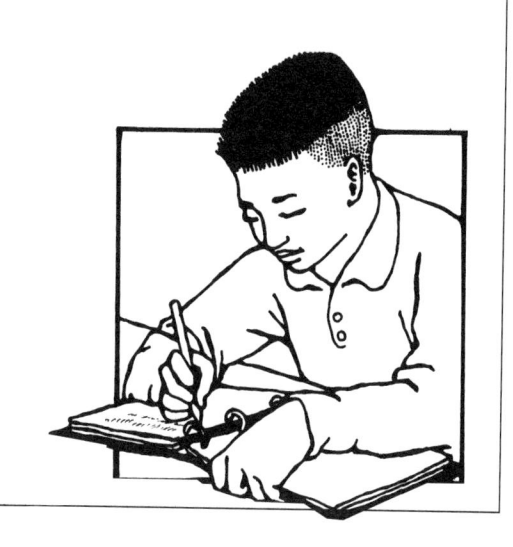

STC / *Food Chemistry* Testing Foods for Starch / **57**

LESSON 4

Record Sheet 4-A

Name: _____

Date: _____

Starch Test for Foods

Pre-Lab Questions

1. What is the nutrient you are testing for? _____

2. What test material are you using to identify the nutrient? _____

3. What is the color of the test material before it is used? _____

Lab

Now test each food for starch. As you complete each test, record your results on the table on the next page. When the table is completed, answer the questions below.

Post-Lab Questions

Using your results, how can you identify a positive test (+) for starch?

_____
_____
_____

Using your results, how can you identify a negative test (–) for starch?

_____
_____
_____

Describe the results of this test on any foods for which the result was not clearly positive or negative: _____
_____
_____

STC / *Food Chemistry*

Record Sheet 4-A (continued)

Name: _____

Date: _____

Starch Test for Foods Table

Test Foods	Prediction: present (+) not present (−) don't know (dk)	Observation of Iodine and Food after Test	First Test Results +, −, dk	Second Test Results +, −, dk
1. Rice				
2. Flour				
3. Apple				
4. Egg white				
5. Peanut				
6. Granola bar				
7. Onion				
8. Coconut				
9.				
10.				

STC / *Food Chemistry*

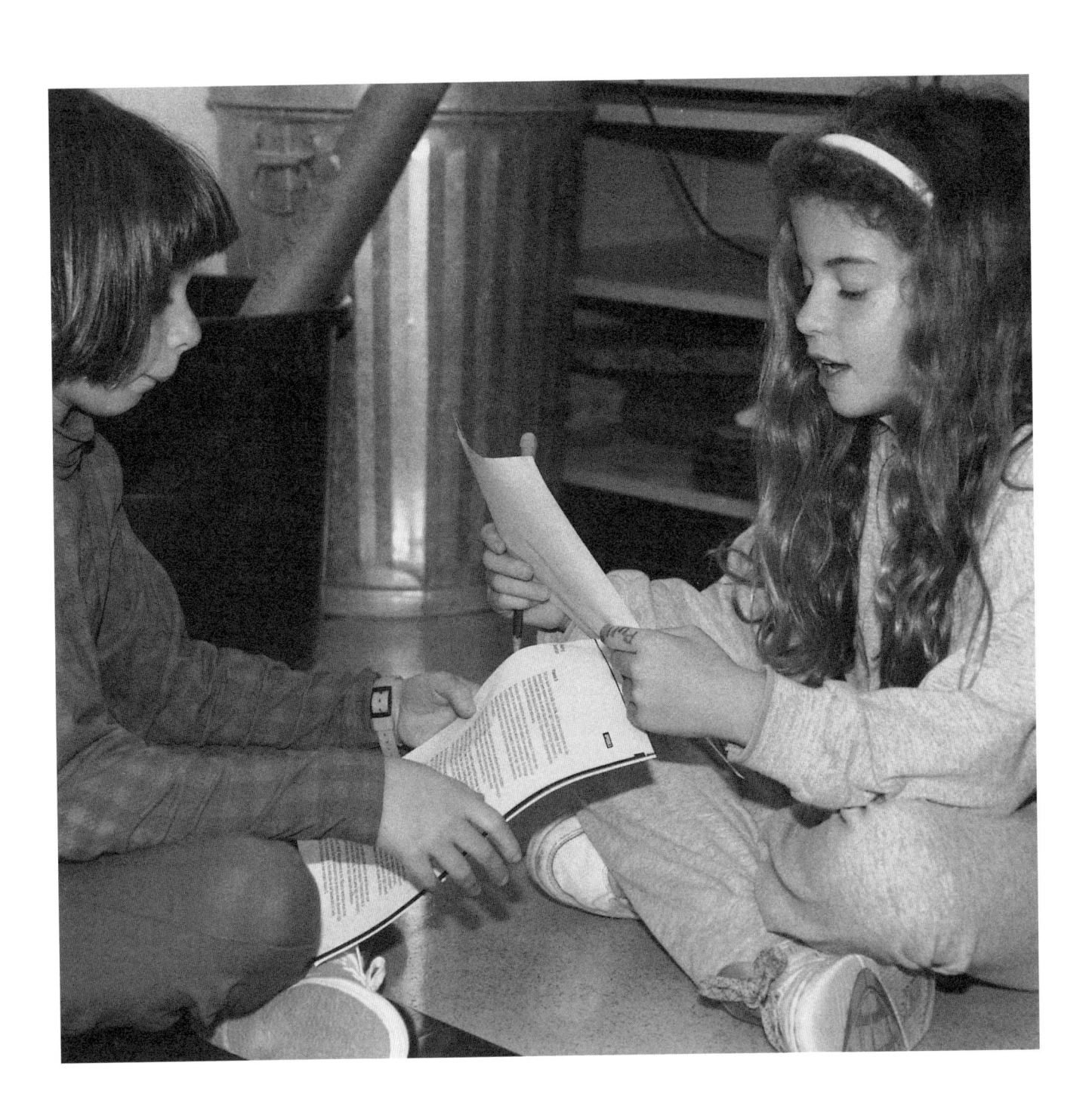

LESSON 5

Learning More about Starch

Overview and Objectives

Students now use what they have learned about how to identify positive and negative tests for starch to interpret and analyze the class's test results. When students discover that results may differ, they retest foods and begin to see that valid conclusions come from repeated testing. Finally, to help them answer questions about starch that cannot be answered through their observation alone, students read about the nutritional value of starch.

- Students analyze and discuss class results from testing foods for starch.
- Students retest foods that provided discrepant results and reexamine their conclusions about which foods contain starch.
- Students read about starch to learn more about how it affects their health.

Background

At the end of this lesson, students will read the first of several **Reading Selections** about how the nutrients studied in this unit are important to their health. (See pg. 65 for "Life Without Starch? It Won't Be Easy!")

In addition, for information on many good books about nutrition, health, and the diets of different cultures around the world, refer to the **Bibliography** in **Appendix B**.

Note: You may want to set up a learning center in which students can continue to do further testing and recording on different foods.

Materials

For each student
1 science notebook
1 **Record Sheet 4-A, Starch Test for Foods** from Lesson 4

For every four students (for retesting, if needed)
1 storage bag containing the following:
    2 lab bags
    1 food bag
    1 liquids bag
4 paper towels

LESSON 5

For the class
> "Class Foods Test Table"
> "Questions We Have about Food" list, from Lesson 1

Preparation

1. Hang the "Questions We Have about Food" list from Lesson 1.
2. Read "Life Without Starch? It Won't Be Easy!" on pg. 65 at the end of this lesson.

Management Tip: Review the **Final Activities** on pg. 63. Depending on your schedule, you may want to assign the reading and/or writing involved as part of a language arts lesson or for homework.

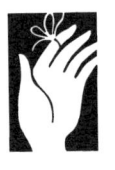

Procedure

1. Begin the lesson by having students describe what they discovered in the last lesson. Then ask the class to take a look at the "Class Foods Test Table."

2. Starting with food No. 1 (rice), ask the following questions:
   - When you tested rice with iodine, what happened?
   - How many positive results were observed?
   - How many negative results were observed?

   Note: At this point, it is important to let children know that their observations are not "right" or "wrong."

3. Moving on to food No. 2 (flour), repeat the questions given above.

4. If test results vary on any of the foods, have students talk about why they think these different results might have occurred. Ask the following questions:
   - Can you think of some reasons why results might differ? (Students may say it is because some experimenters failed to follow directions exactly, they mixed up spoons, or they incorrectly recorded data.)
   - Why is it helpful to look at the whole class's results instead of just one person's results? (Students may say this gives them a lot more data to look at, or that the greater number of test results that agree, the more reliable those results are.)
   - As a class, how can we check our results to determine which foods contain starch?

5. If students do not mention retesting, ask groups to perform a second test on those foods for which results differed. (Students should record "second test" results on their own data tables.) If students need help with the test procedure, refer them back to the **Student Instructions for Testing Foods for Starch** on pg. 18 of the Student Activity Book.

   Management Tip: If several foods need to be retested, you may want to assign each group one of the foods to retest and then share results as a class.

6. When students have finished testing, have the class compare "first test" results with "second test" results. Then ask the following questions:
   - How did first test results compare with second test results?
   - What might students learn from repeating the experiment several times?

Final Activities

1. Have students review the class's "Questions We Have about Food" list. Then, explain that they will be reading about starch and that they should keep these questions in mind and look for information that will help answer some of them.

2. Ask students to read "Life Without Starch? It Won't Be Easy!" on pg. 23 of the Student Activity Book (and pg. 65 of the Teacher's Guide).

3. After they have read about starch, ask students to choose one of the following questions to answer in their science notebooks.

   - Why do people in different parts of the world eat different kinds of starch?
   - Why is starch important to our diet?

Extensions

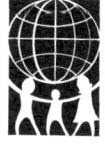

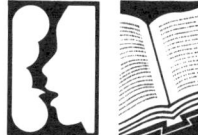

1. Have students make a table showing different countries and the kinds of starch people eat in each.

2. Ask each group to choose one kind of starchy food to study, and make resource books (such as encyclopedias and cookbooks) available. Have each group think of three questions they want to answer about that food to use as a basis for their investigations. Then ask groups to report findings to the class.

3. Students can perform the following experiment to discover for themselves that the body breaks down starch into glucose. Give students the following directions:

   - Put a small piece of white bread in the middle of your tongue.
   - Hold it there for five minutes.
   - How does it taste? (It should taste sweet because enzymes in the mouth break starch down into glucose.)

Assessments

Students have now completed their study of starch and are ready to move on to investigate another kind of carbohydrate—glucose. To evaluate student progress at this time, consider students' laboratory procedures, class discussions, and written observations. The following questions may be helpful.

Lab Procedures
- Are students using the correct number of drops of water and iodine?
- Are students measuring materials with greater accuracy?
- Are students careful to avoid contamination by matching numbers of spoons, foods, and test tray sections? Are they using a different toothpick for each food? Are they wiping the forceps between food preparations?
- Are students willing to retest foods and to reevaluate results?

Discussions
- Do students share their ideas in small group and class discussions?
- Do students listen attentively while others share ideas?
- Do students articulate reasons for discrepant results?

LESSON 5

Written Work

- Do individual students use their tables to organize, record, and interpret data?

- Do individual notebook entries indicate that students understand the test for starch and the need for establishing standards? (You may want to talk with those who have difficulty writing.)

- Did students who retested a food record second test results on their tables?

Management Tip: Lesson 6 requires the advance preparation of glucose test strips for each group. You may want to enlist student helpers for this project during some free time.

Reading Selection

Life Without Starch? It Won't Be Easy!

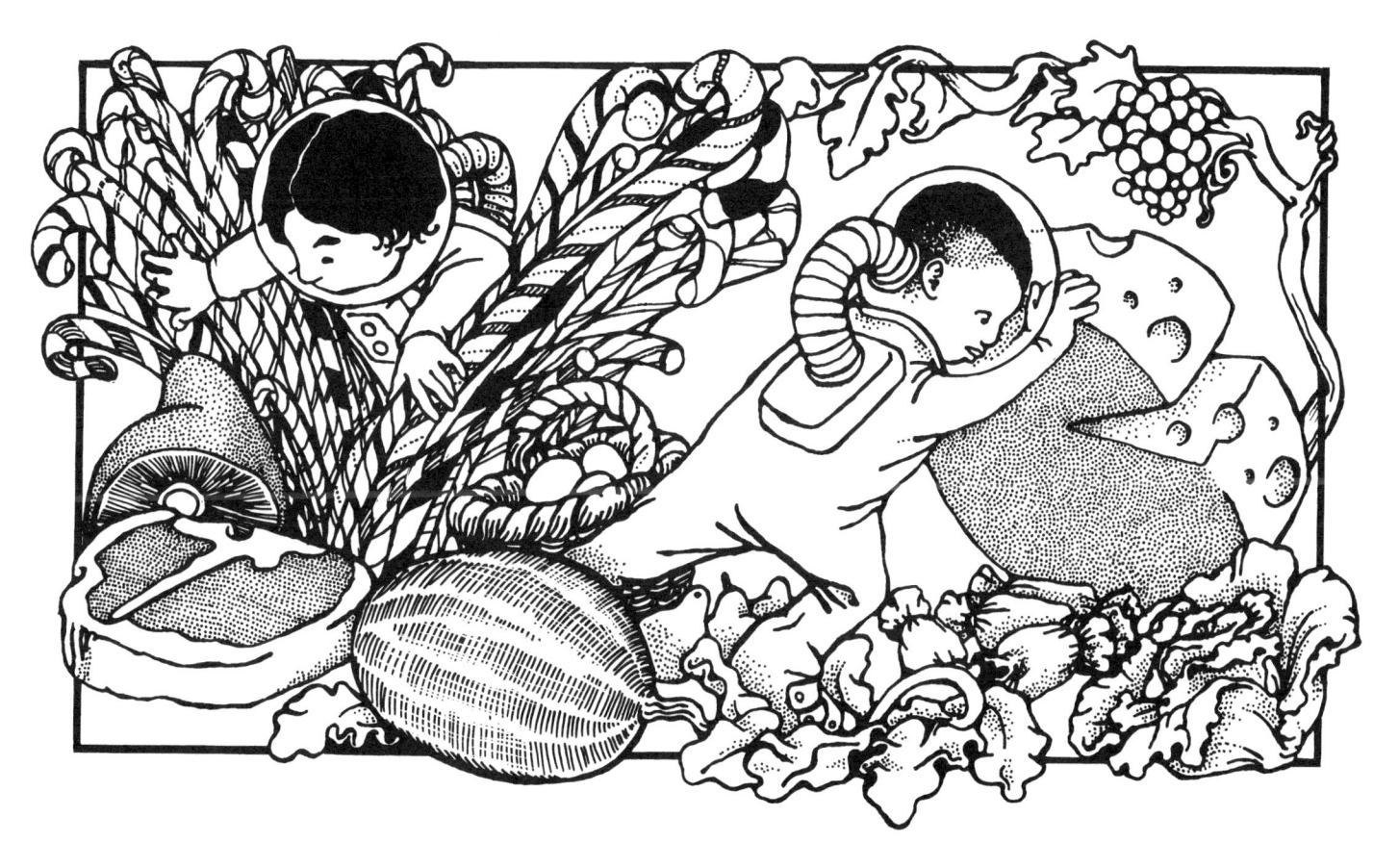

Imagine for a moment that you are an astronaut. You are about to land on a planet that is supposed to have lots of food in a special storehouse. Well, it turns out there is plenty of food. But somehow, none of it contains any starch. As you sort through all that food, you begin to realize that there are no potatoes, rice, bread, beans, or peas. No corn, pasta, or yams. What will you do now?

For one thing, you will have to be extra careful about what other foods you eat.

Starch is the human body's number one source of energy. Without it, the body starts to raid its own energy storehouse; it burns up fat and muscle to get the energy it needs. To prevent that, you will need to eat extra fats and proteins (along with a little sugar) to make up for your lack of starch. What happens if you don't eat extra fats, proteins, and a little sugar? You won't have enough energy even to walk around your space ship. Instead of an explorer, you may end up being an interplanetary couch potato.

LESSON 5

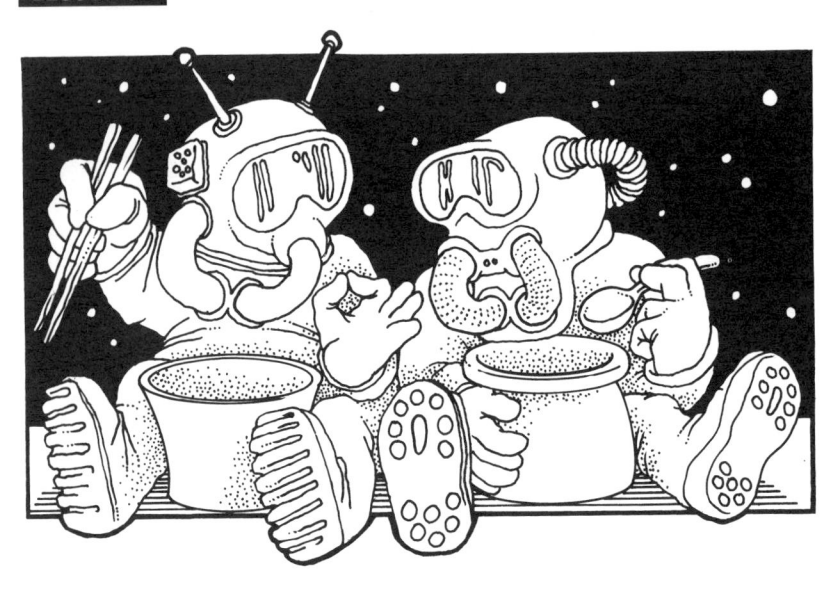

What's Your Favorite Starch?

So, should you call home for supplies? What are your favorite starchy foods? Probably the kind your ancestors liked. For example, if you are an American astronaut, you might ask for bread, beans, or corn. If you are an astronaut from another country, you might ask for special roots, rice, pasta, or beans.

Different people tend to like different sources of starch, depending on the types of starchy vegetables and grains grown in their native countries. In the days before food was traded between countries (and before space travel), people had less of a choice. They simply ate what was around them or what would grow in their soils and climates.

Rice is the principal source of starch on our planet; about half of the world's population depends on it. Rice originally came from India, and today about 90% of the world's rice crop grows in wet areas of the Asian continent. So, naturally, food dishes from this area often contain rice as a main ingredient. If you were a Chinese astronaut, you might ask for rice.

On the other hand, North and South Americans tend to like potatoes. In fact, the potato originally came from Central and South America. Then it was introduced into North America and Europe about the time the New World was settled. Today, potatoes are very popular in food dishes from the United States and Ireland.

Most potatoes are "tubers," so they grow underground. Another tuber that is a vegetable is the water chestnut. Native to the Far East, it is found in Chinese and Japanese dishes. The sweet potato is not a tuber, but we do eat its thick, starchy roots.

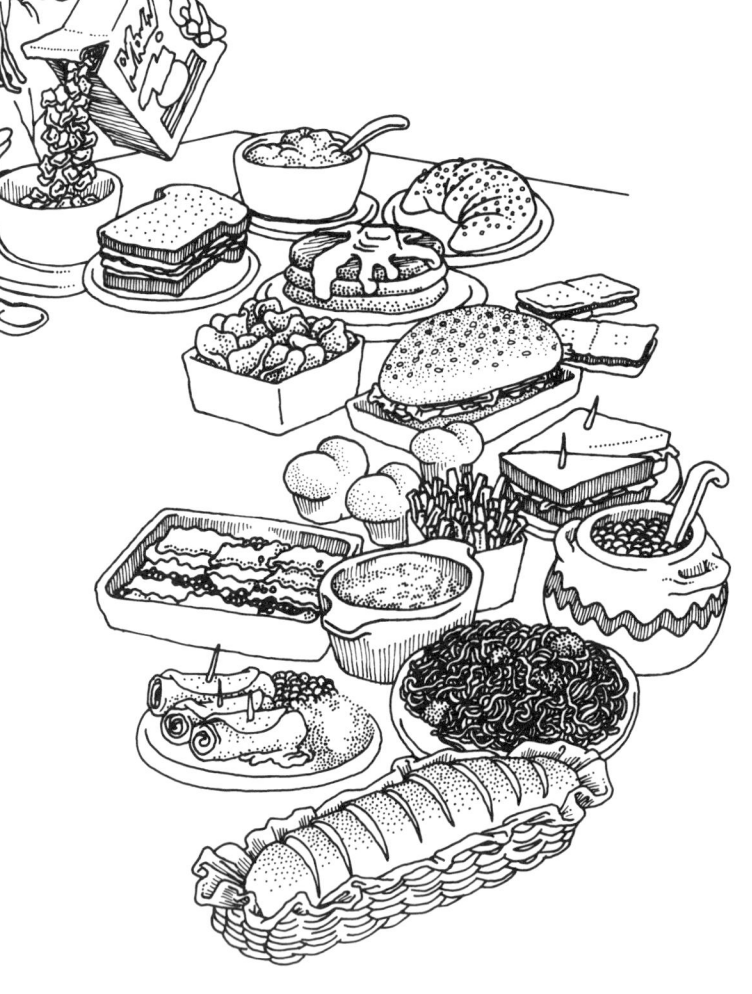

Of course, starch also is found in the wheat, rye, oat, and corn flour that we eat in breads or other products, like pasta. Do you think pasta is an Italian dish? Actually, historians believe pasta noodles were invented in the Orient and brought back to central Europe by the Italian explorer Marco Polo.

Today, many people eat pasta in many different forms. Some athletes eat it the night before the big game as part of a "carbo-loading" plan. (More about that later, in Lesson 8.) What kinds of starch do you eat? Think about it while you're eating dinner tonight.

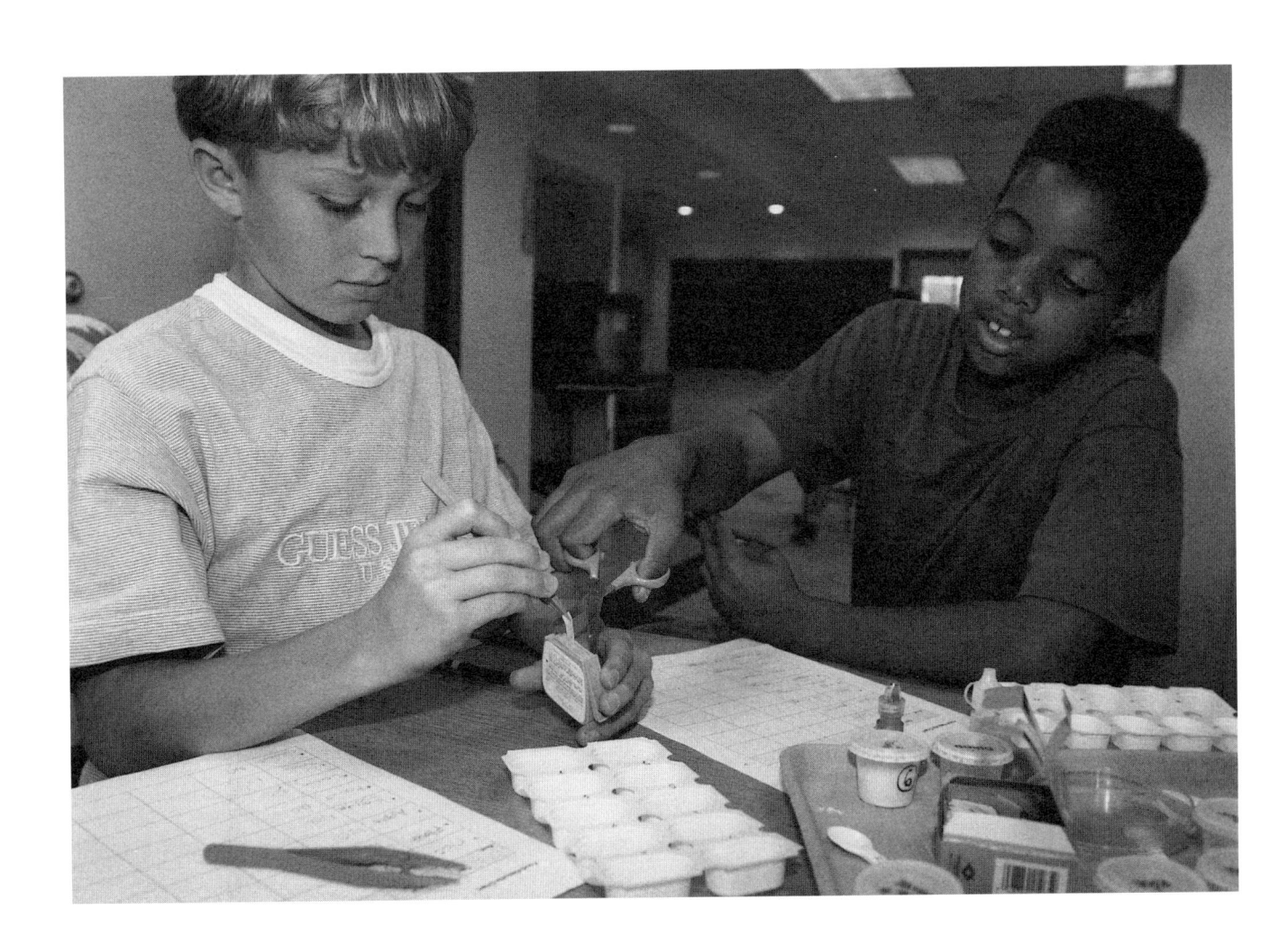

LESSON 6

Testing Liquids for Glucose

Overview and Objectives

For the past three lessons, students have been studying the carbohydrate starch. This lesson introduces students to a new method of testing to identify a second carbohydrate, a simple sugar called glucose. Once again, students will test the five liquids, this time to obtain results that establish a positive and negative test for glucose. Then, in Lesson 7, students will apply to the foods what they have learned about this test and how to interpret results.

- Students make predictions, test liquids for the presence or absence of glucose, and record their results on a **Glucose Test for Liquids Table**.

- Students analyze their test results to establish a positive and negative test for glucose.

- Students record and discuss their findings about the test for glucose.

- Students research and record factual information about glucose.

Background

As mentioned earlier, there are different kinds of carbohydrates, two of which are starches and sugars. And, as Figure 6-1 illustrates, there are several kinds of sugars.

Figure 6-1

How carbohydrates are classified

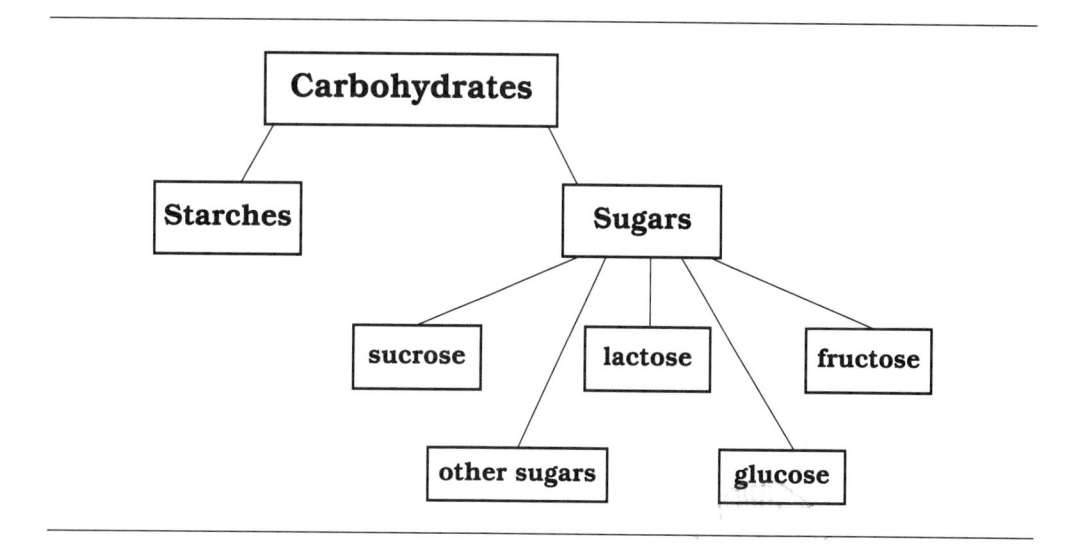

```
                    Carbohydrates
                   /            \
              Starches          Sugars
                             /   |   \
                       sucrose lactose fructose
                            \    |    /
                         other sugars  glucose
```

LESSON 6

Your students may be interested in how these sugars are different. Because sugars differ according to chemical composition—a difficult concept for fifth-graders—you may simply want to point out that there are many kinds of sugar and to share some of the different foods in which they are found (see Figure 6-2).

Figure 6-2

Natural Sources of Some Common Sugars

Sugars	Natural Sources
Glucose	apples, grapes, raisins, bananas, corn
Sucrose	sugar beets, sugar cane
Fructose	apples, pears, peaches
Lactose	milk

In this lesson, students learn a test for a common sugar—glucose. As Figure 6-2 indicates, natural sources of glucose include such fruits as grapes, raisins, and bananas. Soft drinks are another source of glucose familiar to students. Some of the sweet-tasting foods that students are likely to have brought from home will not contain glucose but, rather, another sugar. And some foods, such as apples, do contain glucose (and other types of sugar as well).

Glucose is a major source of energy. Many of the cells in our bodies obtain their energy first from glucose, then from fats, and, finally, from proteins. Because of its small size and simple chemical structure, glucose passes directly into the bloodstream and then to muscles and other cells to provide energy.

As students will learn in this lesson, a simple way to test for glucose is to use glucose test strips. Diabetics use these glucose test papers to determine when their bodies have too much glucose. The papers contain an **enzyme** (a catalyst for chemical changes) that reacts only with glucose, not with any other sugars. In the presence of glucose, the yellow test paper changes to a bright green. This color change results from the enzyme in the paper reacting with the glucose in the substance being tested, as well as with oxygen from the air. The deeper the color, the more glucose is present.

In testing the five liquids, students will discover that the glucose test paper turns green when it is dipped in corn syrup. This establishes a positive test for glucose. With the other four liquids (water, cornstarch, corn oil, and milk), the test paper will not change color. This establishes a negative test for glucose.

Corn syrup is one of the main sweetening agents used in food preparation. When students read food labels in Lesson 15, or on their own at home, they may be able to make this connection.

Students will learn more about glucose and its role in nutrition from both their own research and the **Reading Selection** on pg. 94 in Lesson 8. For more in-depth information on glucose, you may want to look at the **Reading Selection** now.

LESSON 6

Materials

For each student
- 1 science notebook
- 1 **Record Sheet 6-A, Glucose Test for Liquids**

For every four students
- 1 envelope containing 32 glucose test strips
- 1 storage bag containing the following:
  - 2 lab bags
  - 1 food bag
  - 1 liquids bag
- 4 paper towels

For the class
- "Class Liquids Test Table," from Lesson 3, and large marker
- 5 funnels
- 2 clean jars with lids, for mixing 100 ml (3½ oz) quantities of liquid cornstarch and dilute corn syrup
- 1 measuring spoon, 5 ml (1 tsp)
- 1 graduated plastic cup, 100 ml (4½ oz)
- 1 carton of skim milk, 237 ml (½ pt)
- Clear plastic tape
- Newsprint or poster board, or an overhead transparency and pen (see Step 1 in the **Procedure** section)
- Cleanup materials (plastic-lined disposal boxes, paper towels, sponges)
- Soapy water (sink or buckets)
- Clear water (sink or buckets)

Preparation

1. Ask student helpers to put 32 glucose test strips in an envelope for each group of four students. Be sure students use forceps and scissors, since handling the test papers may contaminate them (see Figure 6-3).

   Note: Each pair of students will use six strips today and the other ten strips when they test foods for glucose in Lesson 7.

2. As you did in Lesson 3, prepare the cornstarch and corn syrup according to the following directions:

   - Cornstarch: Mix together 5 ml (1 tsp) of cornstarch and 100 ml (3½ oz) of tap water.

   - Corn syrup: Mix together 5 ml (1 tsp) of corn syrup and 100 ml (3½ oz) of tap water.

Figure 6-3

Using forceps

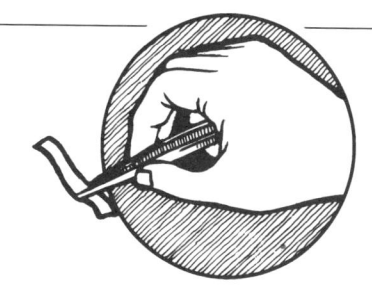

LESSON 6

3. Obtain 237 ml (½ pt) of skim milk.

4. Have student helpers refill the dropper bottles containing water, cornstarch, corn oil, corn syrup, and milk. Remind them to use a different funnel for each liquid except water.

5. Make one copy of **Record Sheet 6-A, Glucose Test for Liquids** for each student.

6. Post the "Class Liquids Test Table" from Lesson 3.

Procedure

1. Begin the lesson by asking students briefly to discuss what they know about sugar. Record students' ideas on newsprint or an overhead transparency. Or, ask students quickly to record ideas in their notebooks.

2. Next, explain how students will test for a type of sugar called glucose using the same five liquids they used in Lesson 3.

3. Distribute **Record Sheet 6-A, Glucose Test for Liquids**. Review the pre- and post-lab questions and ask students to fill in the table with the names of the five test liquids. Suggest that they refer back to their liquids tables for the starch test (**Record Sheet 3-A**) to help remember the liquids and the correct order in which they should be listed and tested.

4. Now use forceps to hold up a strip of glucose test paper. Explain how the paper is used as a chemical test material for detecting glucose, and how it will undergo a chemical reaction if glucose is present.

5. Next ask students how they might use glucose test papers to test the liquids. Encourage them to think about their experiences in Lesson 3 when they tested the five liquids for starch.

6. Then have students write on the table on **Record Sheet 6-A** their predictions about which liquids will or will not contain glucose.

7. Review the **Student Instructions for Testing Liquids for Glucose** on pg. 75 of this guide and on pg. 30 of the Student Activity Book.

   Note: Remind students to wipe the forceps carefully with a paper towel after they place each test strip into a liquid.

8. Then have one person from each group pick up the following: the group's storage bag, one envelope containing the glucose test papers, clear plastic tape, and four paper towels. Let students get to work.

9. At cleanup time, have students follow the directions below (also found on pg. 28 of the Student Activity Book):

   - Put the envelope with the unused glucose test papers in the storage bag to use in Lesson 7.
   - Empty and rinse out the dropper bottles of cornstarch, corn syrup, and milk.
   - Wash, rinse, and dry the forceps and return them to the lab bag.
   - Wipe the test trays with paper towels, wash and rinse them out, and then wipe them again.
   - Place the five dropper bottles back into the liquids bag.
   - Return all the materials to the storage bag.
   - Return the storage bag to the storage area.

Final Activities

1. Have students look at the "Class Liquids Test Table" from Lesson 3. Once again, ask a member from each group to come up to the table and write his or her group's test results (+ or –) for each liquid.

2. Then, starting with water, ask students to describe in detail what happened to the glucose test paper with each liquid.

3. Have students discuss their conclusions about this test by asking questions such as:

    - Which liquids contain glucose?
    - Which liquids do not contain glucose?
    - How do you know?
    - How do your results compare to your predictions?

4. Discuss any differing results. Ask students to repeat the test to see if they get the same results the second time. Make sure they record the second set of results on **Record Sheet 6-A**. Be sure to save the "Class Liquids Test Table" for use in Lessons 9 and 12.

    Note: If there is not time to retest now, have students do so at a convenient time later in the day.

5. Ask students to describe in their notebooks which liquids contain glucose and which do not, as well as their reasons for saying so.

6. Ask each student to research and record two interesting facts about glucose, either as homework or at school during library time. Ask them to be prepared to share the information they discover about glucose before they test the foods in Lesson 7.

Extensions

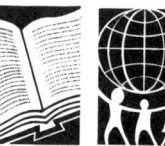

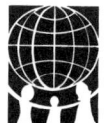

1. Have students research other sugars, such as sucrose or fructose.

2. Have students make a map showing places in the world where plant sources of sugar are grown.

3. Invite a nurse or doctor to visit the class and explain how diabetics use the glucose test papers.

4. Have each group of four students make a poster that presents the information they found about glucose. As a class, compare posters to see how many unique facts students have learned.

Assessments

This is the first of three lessons in the glucose test cycle. During this cycle look for growth in the following areas.

Lab Procedures
- Do students follow the instructions for performing the glucose test?
- Are students careful not to contaminate materials?
- Is the cleanup becoming routine?

LESSON 6

Discussions

- Do students accurately discuss the results of their investigations?
- Can students relate experiences with the starch test to experiences with the glucose test?
- During the **Final Activities** of these lessons, can students draw some conclusions about the liquids and foods that do and do not contain glucose?
- At the end of the cycle, can students discuss why some sweet-tasting foods did not test positive for glucose?

Written Work

- Do students record their test data on the Record Sheets as they observe results, rather than after they have finished testing?
- Do students identify and describe liquids and foods which do and do not contain glucose?
- When students compare starch and glucose, do they include information from their notebooks, tables, research, and reading selections?
- Do the Venn diagrams indicate an understanding of some ways in which starch and glucose are similar? Some ways in which they are different?

Student Instructions for Testing Liquids for Glucose

1. Answer pre-lab questions 1 and 2 on **Record Sheet 6-A**.

2. With the forceps, place one glucose test paper in each of the five numbered sections in the test tray. Tape one test paper on the top of the table on **Record Sheet 6-A** to use as the control.

3. Then answer pre-lab question 3 on **Record Sheet 6-A**.

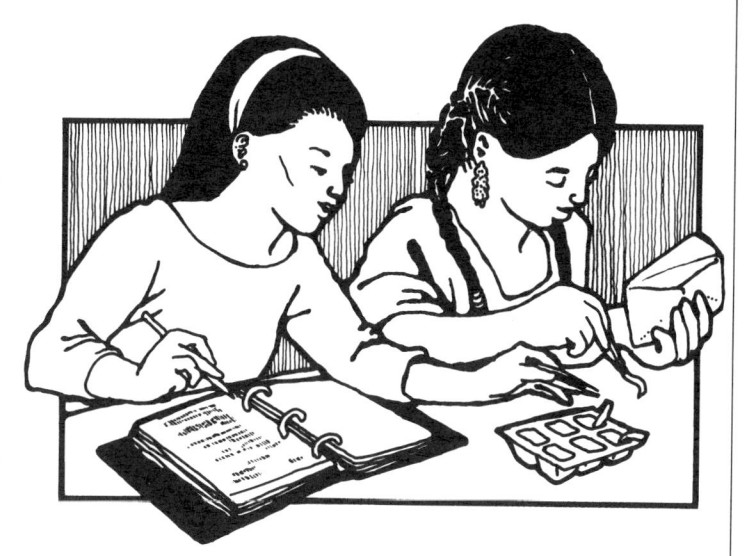

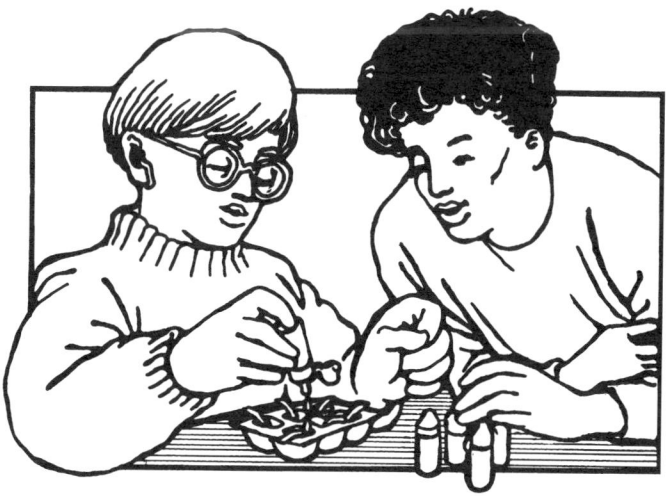

4. Put two drops of the first liquid (water) directly on the test paper in section 1.

5. Wait a few seconds, and then observe the color of the paper. How does it compare to the control? Discuss this with your group and record your observation on the table on **Record Sheet 6-A**. Tape the test paper on your Record Sheet next to the word "Water."

6. Next, put two drops of the second liquid (cornstarch) directly on the test paper in section 2. Again, discuss observations with your teammates, and record them on your Record Sheet. Tape the test paper there, too, next to the word "Cornstarch."

7. Repeat this process with corn syrup, corn oil, and milk. Make sure the numbers on the dropper bottles match the numbers of your tray sections.

8. With your group, decide which liquid(s) tested positive (+) for glucose and which tested negative (−). Record your decisions on the table on your Record Sheet.

9. Complete the two post-lab questions.

10. Clean up.

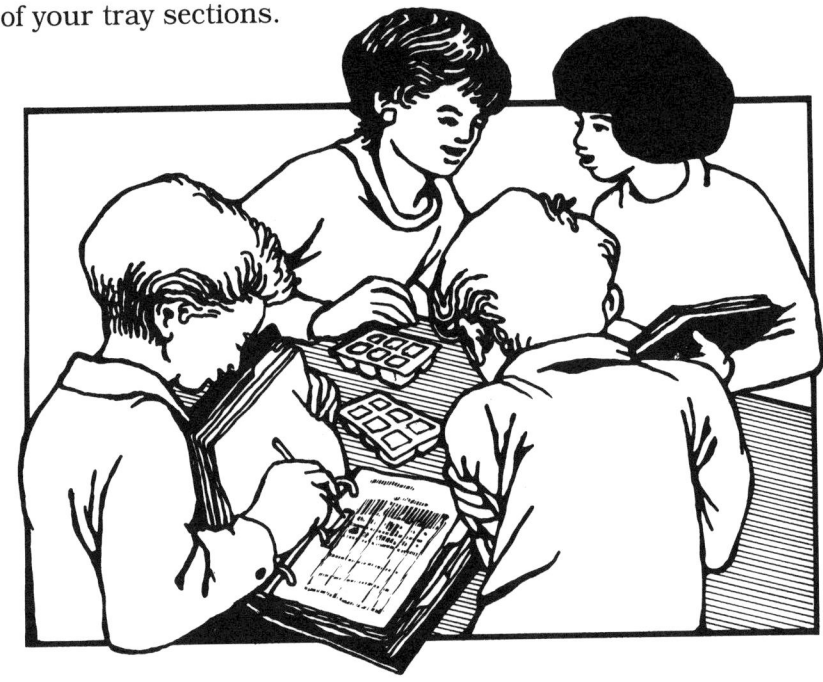

Record Sheet 6-A　　　　　　　Name: _____

　　　　　　　　　　　　　　　　Date: _____

Glucose Test for Liquids

Pre-Lab Questions

1. What is the nutrient you are testing for? _____
   _____

2. What test material are you using to identify the nutrient? _____
   _____

3. What is the color of the test material before it is used? _____
   _____

Lab

Now test each liquid for glucose. As you complete each test, record your results on the table on the next page. When the table is completed, answer the questions below.

Post-Lab Questions

Using your results, how can you identify a positive test (+) for glucose?

_____

_____

_____

Using your results, how can you identify a negative test (–) for glucose?

_____

_____

_____

STC / *Food Chemistry*

LESSON 6

Record Sheet 6-A (continued)

Name: _____

Date: _____

Glucose Test for Liquids Table

Test Liquids	Prediction: present (+) not present (−) don't know (dk)	Observation of Glucose Test Paper after Test	First Test Results +, −, dk	Second Test Results +, −, dk
1.				
2.				
3.				
4.				
5.				

STC / *Food Chemistry*

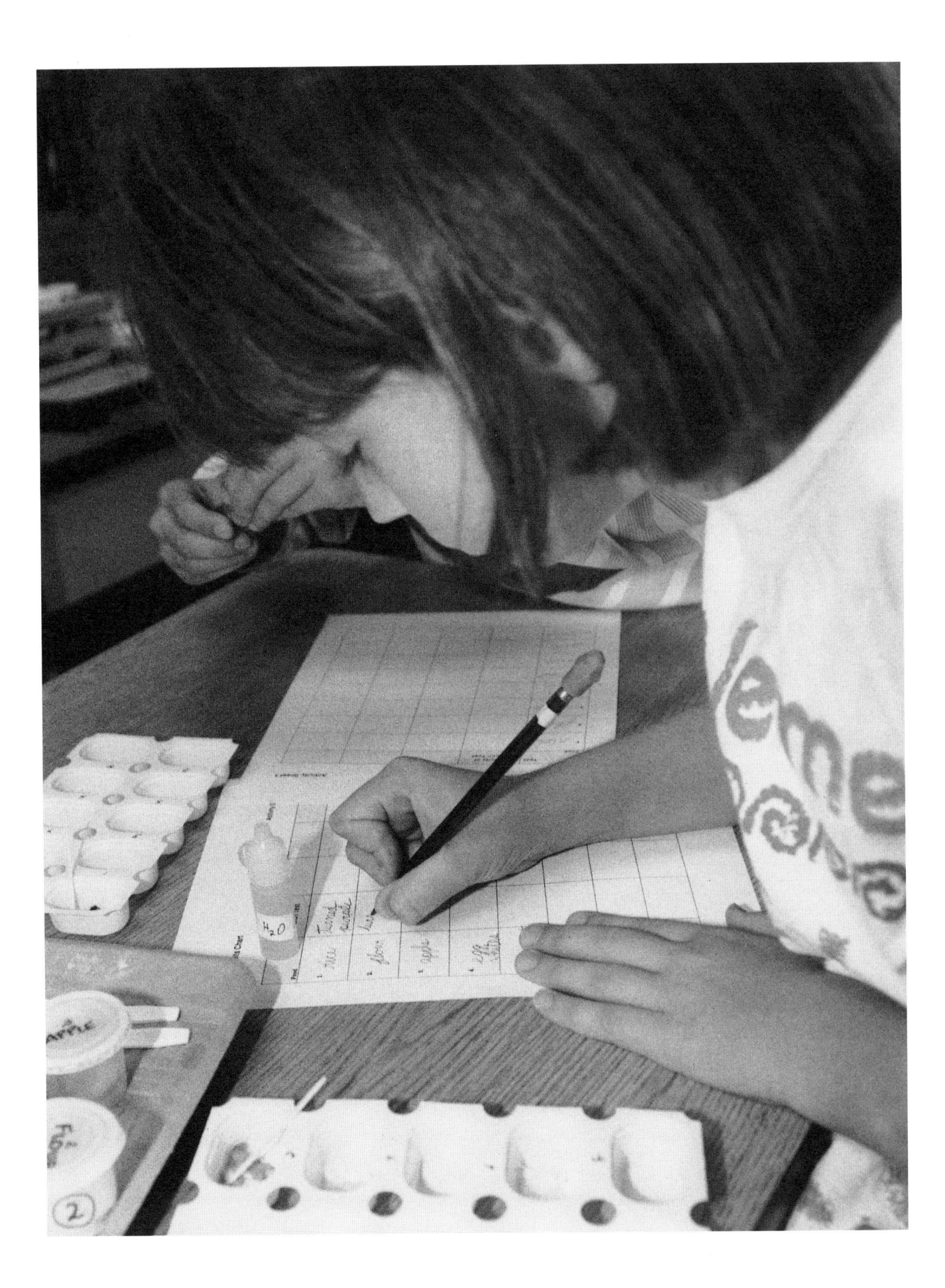

LESSON 7

Testing Foods for Glucose

Overview and Objectives

In Lesson 6, students learned to use a chemically treated paper to test for the presence or absence of glucose. In this investigation, they apply the test for glucose to identify the foods that do and do not contain this simple sugar. Throughout the testing process, students are likely to observe a range of reactions. They will be introduced to a number of concepts—that test results are not always clearly positive or clearly negative, that different foods vary in the quantity of glucose they contain, and that foods might contain more than one nutrient. In coming lessons, tests for proteins and fats will help to reinforce these concepts.

- Students share with the class what they have learned about glucose through individual research.

- Students make and record predictions about the foods they think do and do not contain glucose.

- Students apply the glucose test to their foods and compare the range of test results with their predictions.

- In their notebooks, students record discoveries and questions about glucose.

Background

In this lesson, the test for glucose will produce varying results based on the amount of glucose present in each food. In general, you can expect the apple and granola bar to test positive for glucose. Other foods may also have slight positive reactions, indicating the presence of very small amounts of glucose.

As students encounter varying test results, discuss with them how to interpret a range of reactions and help them understand that test results are not always definitive. The glucose test strips come with a color table that might help the students judge their test results (see the **Student Instructions for Testing Foods for Glucose** on pg. 85). Students should also be encouraged to remember that repeating tests can help them validate results.

Note that because the test papers for this glucose test were designed primarily for use by diabetics, they do not register the presence of sugars other than glucose, such as those found in most baked goods and cereals. Since students know that such foods contain sugar, they may be puzzled if they test them and the results are not positive.

STC / *Food Chemistry*

LESSON 7

In addition to the research they have done about glucose, your students will learn more about glucose and how it relates to nutrition in the **Reading Selection** in Lesson 8 (pg. 94).

Materials

For each student
- 1 science notebook
- 1 **Record Sheet 7-A, Glucose Test for Foods**
- 1 completed **Record Sheet 4-A, Starch Test for Foods**, from Lesson 4
- 1 completed **Record Sheet 6-A, Glucose Test for Liquids**, from Lesson 6

For every four students
- 1 storage bag containing the following:
  - 1 envelope with 20 glucose test strips
  - 1 food bag
  - 2 lab bags
  - 1 liquids bag
- 4 paper towels

For the class
- "Class Foods Test Table"
- Color tables for glucose test strips
- Clear plastic tape
- Cleanup materials (2 plastic-lined disposal boxes, sponges, paper towels)
- Soapy water (sink or buckets)
- Clear water (sink or buckets)

Preparation

1. If necessary, have a student refill the dropper bottles of water that were used in Lesson 6.

2. Make one copy of **Record Sheet 7-A, Glucose Test for Foods** for each student.

Procedure

1. Begin by asking students to share the information they have researched about glucose since the last lesson. You may want to have students record this information on a class list.

2. Then ask students how they might apply what they learned from testing the liquids for glucose to determine if the foods contain glucose.

3. Distribute **Record Sheet 7-A, Glucose Test for Foods** and briefly discuss the pre- and post-lab questions. Ask students to fill in the names of their test foods in the right order in the first column. They may want to look back at their starch test tables for foods from Lesson 4 to help them remember the foods and the correct order in which they should be listed and tested.

4. Now ask students to predict for each food whether glucose is present or not and to write the predictions on their tables. Again, emphasize that a prediction is not a test and there is no right or wrong.

5. Briefly review the **Student Instructions for Testing Foods for Glucose** on pg. 85 in this guide and pg. 36 of the Student Activity Book. Remind students to wipe the forceps carefully with a paper towel after each use with a different food.

   Note: Foods need time to become soaked or dissolved in water prior to the glucose test. Specifically, the rice needs to be soaked. This can take as long as five minutes, depending on the rice used. Discuss this with the class so that they do not dip the glucose strip in water that does not yet contain nutrients from the food.

6. Have a member from each group pick up the following: the group's storage bag, clear plastic tape, and four paper towels. Then, let the class get to work.

7. At cleanup time, have students follow the directions below (also found on pg. 34 of the Student Activity Book):

   - Discard the contents of the test trays and the used toothpicks into the plastic-lined disposal boxes.
   - Put the correct lids securely on the food cups.
   - Wipe the spoons with a paper towel and return the food cups and spoons to the food bag.
   - Return the box of toothpicks and dropper bottles of water to the liquids bag.
   - Wash the test trays in soapy water, rinse them in clear water, and wipe them dry.
   - Wash, rinse, and dry the forceps, and return them and the test trays to the lab bag.
   - Return all materials to the storage bag.

8. After they have cleaned up, ask one student from each group to record that group's glucose test results on the "Class Foods Test Table." Let students know they will discuss these results in the next lesson.

   Management Tip: In Lesson 8, the class may retest foods for which test results were discrepant. You will need to prepare glucose strips for this retesting.

Final Activities

1. Ask students to write a few sentences in their notebooks answering the following questions:

   - What did you discover during this investigation?
   - Which of the foods that you predicted would contain glucose tested positive?
   - Which of the foods that you predicted would not contain glucose tested positive?
   - Which of the foods contain both glucose and starch?
   - What questions do you have about glucose?

2. When students are finished writing, have them share answers in a class discussion.

LESSON 7

Extensions

1. If students test additional foods for glucose, suggest that they do they following:

   - Arrange the test papers in order to show which indicate the most to least glucose.
   - Tape the glucose test papers to an index card.
   - Label the card with the name of each food.
   - Put the cards on a class bulletin board with pictures of the foods tested.

   Note: Bear in mind that the colors on the glucose test strips may change or fade shortly after foods are tested for glucose.

2. Have students predict what will happen if they retest the foods for glucose but do not first add drops of water. Then have them retest without the water. Remember that students will need to record their results. Hold a class discussion about the results.

3. Have students create "shape" poems about their favorite foods containing glucose or another kind of sugar (see Figure 7-1). The lines of the poem will create the shape of the food.

Figure 7-1

Sample shape poem

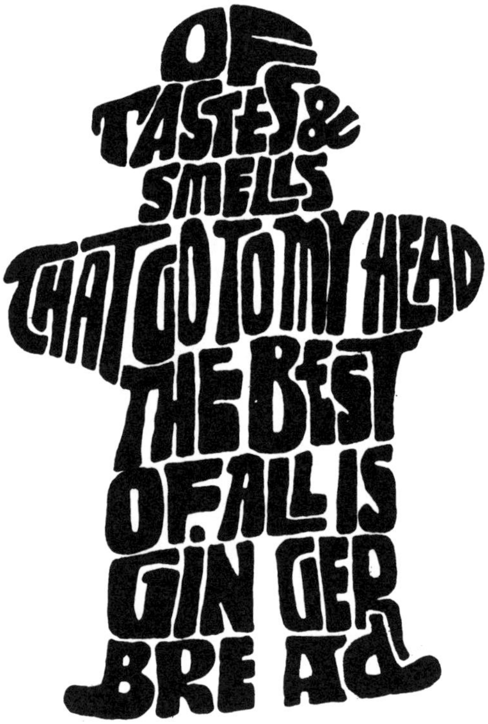

Student Instructions for Testing Foods for Glucose

1. Answer pre-lab questions 1 and 2 on **Record Sheet 7-A**.

2. As with the starch test, some foods need preparation before testing. You and your partner may use your fingers to shell the peanut since you will not be touching the actual food. (Touching the test food with your fingers may contaminate the foods.) Use your forceps to place a shelled peanut or two and small portions of dried apple and granola into their matching numbered sections of the test tray. Then, also with forceps, do the following:
   - Tear the apple into small pieces.
   - Remove the peanut's papery skin. Hold down the peanut with forceps and have your partner use the other forceps to crumble the kernel.
   - Crumble a small piece of the granola bar.

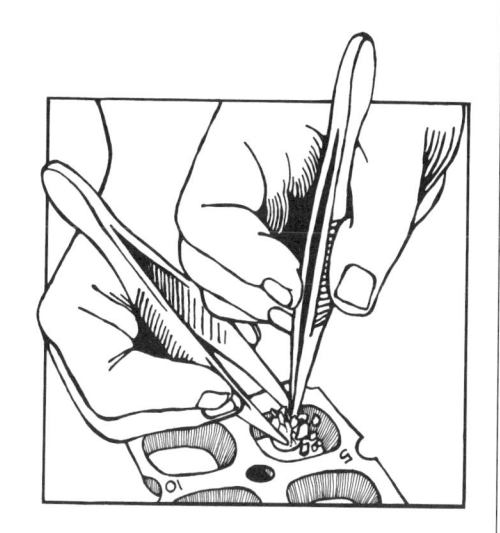

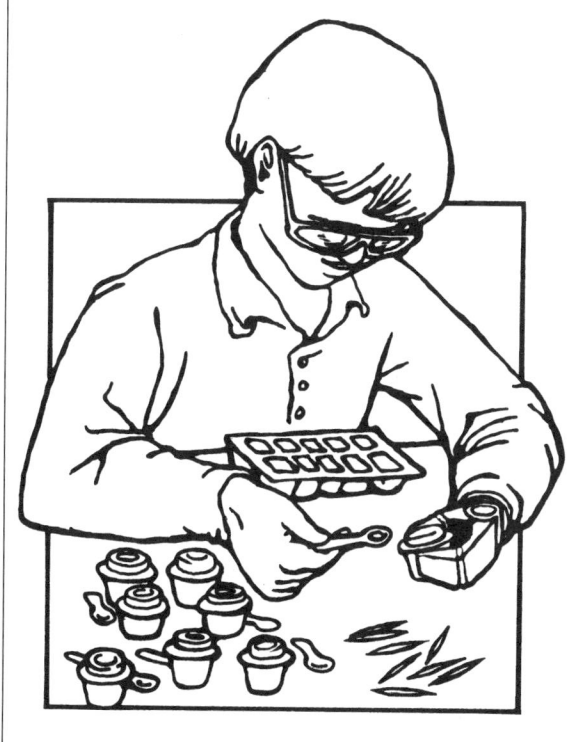

3. Put one spoonful of each of the other foods into your test tray. Make sure the number of each spoon matches the number of the food and the test tray section you place it in.

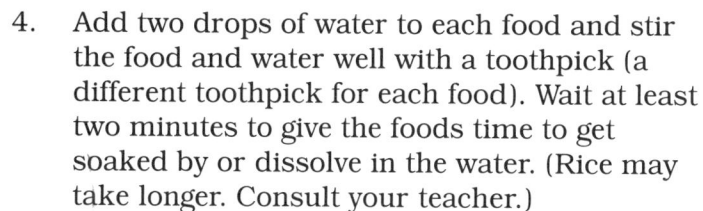

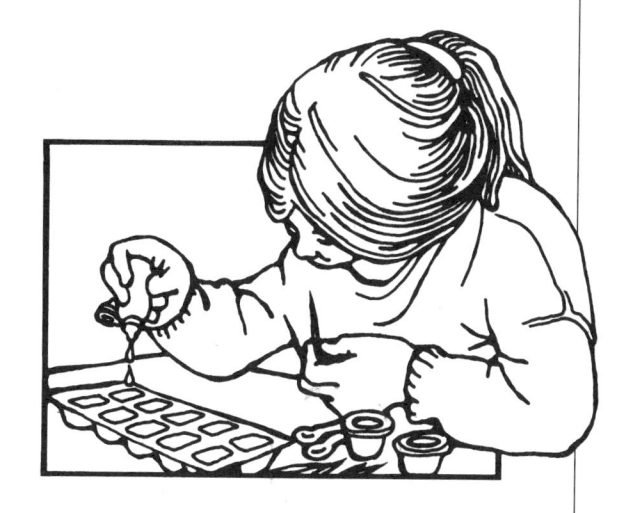

4. Add two drops of water to each food and stir the food and water well with a toothpick (a different toothpick for each food). Wait at least two minutes to give the foods time to get soaked by or dissolve in the water. (Rice may take longer. Consult your teacher.)

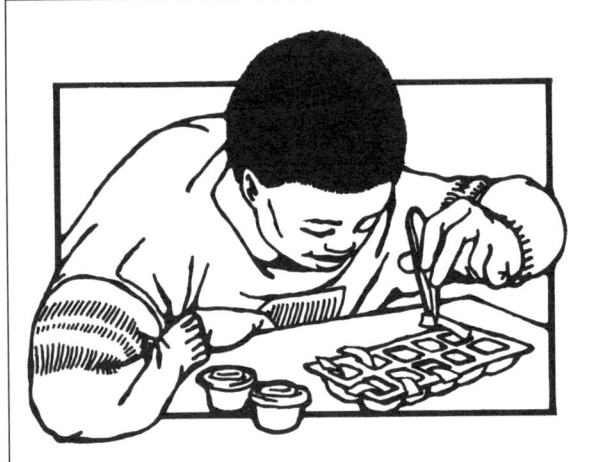

5. Use the forceps to put one strip of glucose test paper in each tray section with the food and water mixture. Make sure at least half of every glucose test paper is wet.

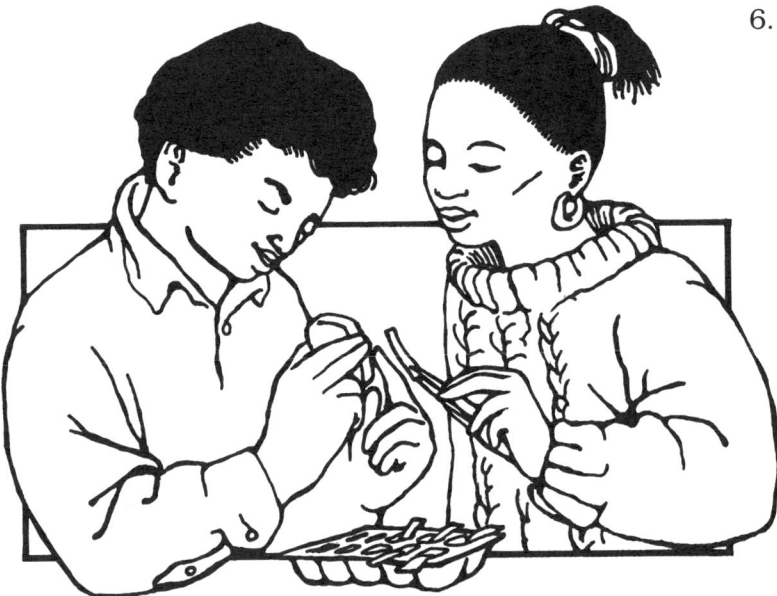

6. Wait a few seconds and then observe the color of the paper in tray section 1. How does it compare to the control paper you taped to **Record Sheet 6-A**? For each result, also check the color table for the glucose test paper to see if glucose is present. If so, how much? Share your observations with your teammates.

7. Record your observations for the first food on **Record Sheet 7-A**. Tape the test paper on the Record Sheet next to the name of the first food.

8. Repeat this process for the other foods. Be sure to tape each glucose test paper on your Record Sheet next to the name of its food.

9. With your group, decide which food(s) tested positive (+) and which tested negative (−). Record your decisions on your Record Sheet.

10. Complete the post-lab questions.

11. Now follow your cleanup instructions.

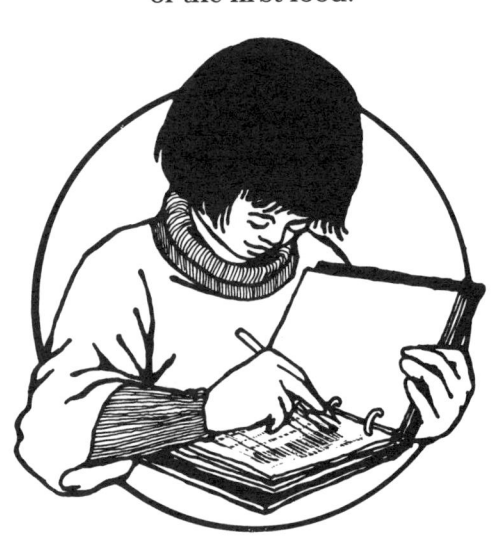

Record Sheet 7-A   Name: _____

                                        Date: _____

LESSON 7

Glucose Test for Foods

Pre-Lab Questions

1. What is the nutrient you are testing for? _____
   _____

2. What test material are you using to identify the nutrient? _____
   _____

3. What is the color of the test material before it is used? _____
   _____

Lab

Now test each liquid for glucose. As you complete each test, record your results on the table on the next page. When the table is completed, answer the questions below.

Post-Lab Questions

Using your results, how can you identify a positive test (+) for glucose?
_____
_____

Using your results, how can you identify a negative test (−) for glucose?
_____
_____

Describe the results of this test on any food for which the result was not clearly positive or negative. _____
_____

STC / *Food Chemistry*

LESSON 7

Record Sheet 7-A (continued)

Name: _____

Date: _____

Glucose Test for Foods Table

Test Foods	Prediction: present (+) not present (−) don't know (dk)	Observation of Glucose Test Paper after Test	First Test Results +, −, dk	Second Test Results +, −, dk
1.				
2.				
3.				
4.				
5.				
6.				
7.				
8.				
9.				
10.				

STC / *Food Chemistry*

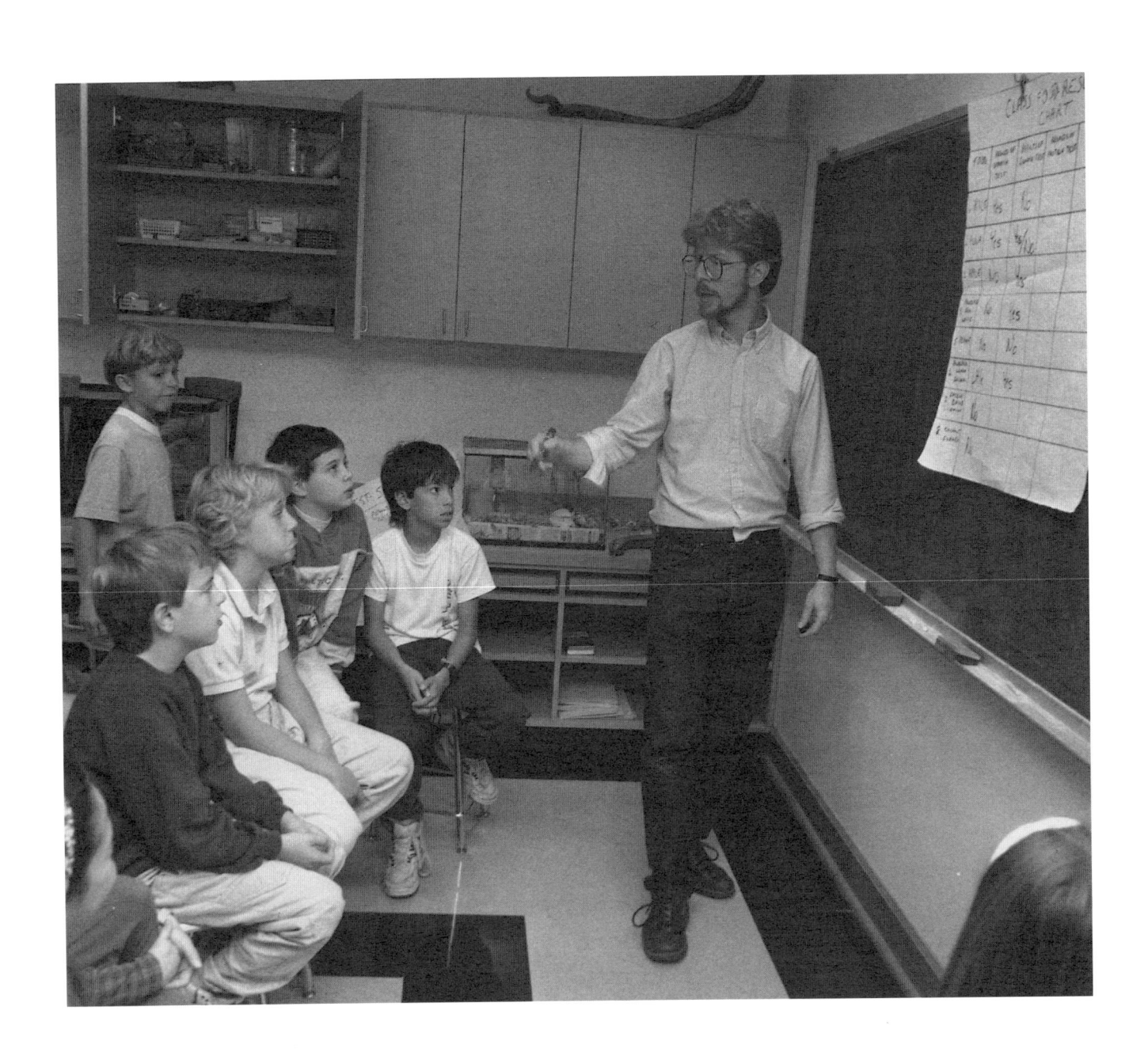

| LESSON 8 | **Learning More about Glucose** |

Overview and Objectives

Students now have learned to test foods for two kinds of carbohydrates—starch and glucose. This lesson helps students draw some conclusions about how starch and glucose are alike and different. After groups compare their results from the glucose test, they consider why results for some foods may differ and retest those foods to validate test results. Students then read about the nutritional value of glucose.

- Students analyze and discuss their results from testing the foods for glucose.
- Students retest foods for which there were discrepant results among groups.
- Students read and write about the role glucose plays in their diets.
- Each student uses a Venn diagram to compare starch with glucose.

Background

Students now have tested foods for both starch and glucose. But they will need some help understanding the differences between these two kinds of carbohydrates, particularly in terms of the roles they play in diet and human health.

Both the Venn diagrams students will create and the **Reading Selection** on pg. 94 at the end of this lesson will help the class to draw clearer distinctions between starch and glucose. (For more information on Venn diagrams, see pg. 6.) In addition, the Reading Selection will show some ways in which the two kinds of carbohydrates may relate to students' own lives.

Materials

For each student
- 1 science notebook
- 1 **Record Sheet 7-A, Glucose Test for Foods** from Lesson 7

For every four students (for retesting, if needed)
- 1 storage bag containing the following:
    - 1 food bag
    - 2 lab bags
    - 1 liquids bag
- Extra glucose test papers

STC / *Food Chemistry*

LESSON 8

For the class
- 1 sheet of newsprint or poster board and large marker
- "Class Foods Test Table," from previous lessons
- "Questions We Have about Foods" list, from Lesson 1

Preparation

1. Post the "Class Foods Test Table."

2. Copy the following questions onto the sheet of newsprint:
   - What are some foods that contain both starch and glucose?
   - Why are starch and glucose important in our diets?
   - If you were running a 50-yard dash tomorrow, what kind of carbohydrate would you eat and why?
   - If you were going on a ten-mile hike tomorrow, what kind of carbohydrate would you eat and why?

3. Read "Low on Energy? Here's What to Eat," on pg. 94.

   Management Tip: You may want to assign the reading and/or the writing portion of the **Final Activities** as part of a language arts lesson or for homework.

4. Prepare enough glucose test papers for any retesting required.

Procedure

1. Ask students to describe what they learned about the presence or absence of glucose in their foods. Students may want to refer to their notebooks and **Record Sheet 7-A, Glucose Test for Foods**.

2. Using the "Class Foods Test Table," hold a class discussion to analyze test results. The following questions will be helpful in guiding the discussion:
   - Which foods tested positive for glucose? How do you know?
   - Which foods tested negative for glucose? How do you know?
   - Which foods had results that were less clear?
   - For which foods did groups obtain different test results?
   - What might you do to check the accuracy of these results?

3. Allow time for students to check their results by retesting foods for which results differed. Remind them to record these results in the "second test" column on their foods tables. Depending on the number of different results, you may want to assign each group one food to test.

Final Activities

1. Let students know they will learn more about glucose and starch from reading "Low on Energy? Here's What to Eat," on pg. 41 of the Student Activity Book (and on pg. 94 of this guide).

2. Post the list of four questions you prepared earlier for students to refer to in the following activity.

Figure 8-1

Sample of completed Venn diagram

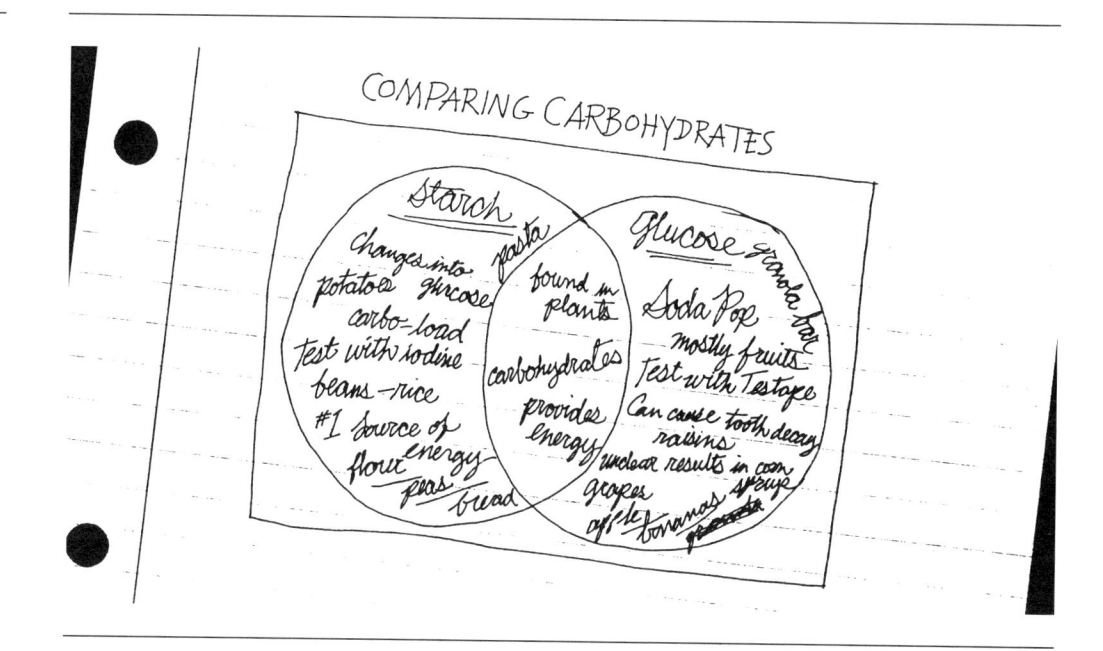

COMPARING CARBOHYDRATES

Starch: changes into glucose, potatoes, carbo-load, test with iodine, beans-rice, #1 source of energy, flour, peas, pasta

Both (center): found in plants, carbohydrates, provides energy, bread

Glucose: granola bar, Soda Pop, mostly fruits, Test with Testape, Can cause tooth decay, raisins, unclear results in corn syrup, grapes, apples, bananas

---

3. Ask each student to draw a Venn diagram in his or her notebook comparing the two kinds of carbohydrates. Encourage students to use their record sheets, notebook entries, and reading selections as sources of information. Also explain that they may find it helpful to keep in mind the list of four questions. (See Figure 8-1 for a sample of a completed Venn diagram.)

   Note: Remind students to add any new questions to the "Questions We Have about Food" list.

Extensions

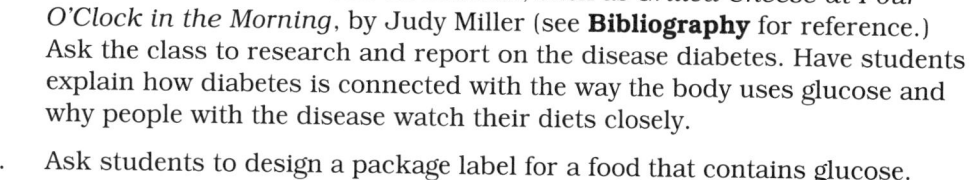

1. Have students read a book on diabetes, such as *Grilled Cheese at Four O'Clock in the Morning*, by Judy Miller (see **Bibliography** for reference.) Ask the class to research and report on the disease diabetes. Have students explain how diabetes is connected with the way the body uses glucose and why people with the disease watch their diets closely.

2. Ask students to design a package label for a food that contains glucose.

3. Plan a lunch featuring foods that contain starch and glucose.

4. Bananas are a natural source of glucose. Challenge students to estimate what percentage of a banana they actually eat. Then have them figure out the cost of just the edible portion.

Assessments

To help you assess student growth at this time, you may want to refer back to the **Assessments** section on pg. 73 of Lesson 6.

LESSON 8

Reading Selection

Low on Energy? Here's What to Eat

In Lesson 5, we pretended to be astronauts stranded on a planet with no starchy foods. We realized that we could not remain active for very long without starches, because we get most of our energy when our bodies break starches down into glucose. So we ordered a cargo ship full of starchy foods such as potatoes, rice, breads, pasta, corn, peas, and beans.

But now the ship is late. What are we going to do? How will we get glucose for energy if not from eating starches? Although our bodies will continue to make glucose on their own, they will eventually need more, from food.

Would corn syrup be a good source? After all, it's one of the few foods in which glucose is the only sugar. But if we were to eat glucose alone, we wouldn't get many of the other things that our bodies need to stay healthy. So eating only corn syrup or other foods that are high in glucose is not the answer.

We could always get temporary energy by drinking soft drinks, since many of them are sweetened with corn syrup and fructose. (Fructose is another kind of sugar found mainly in fruits.) However, we would have to drink a lot of this sweet stuff, which probably would make us sick. Also, these sugary drinks don't provide us with any of the other nutrients our bodies need to grow and repair themselves.

That's not all. We would probably develop serious health problems if we continued to eat too much sugar. For one thing, eating too much glucose and other sugars is a major cause of tooth decay. Also, too much glucose causes our

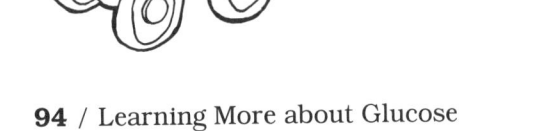

94 / Learning More about Glucose

a steady source of energy. We will probably start eating starchy foods as soon as possible, and we'll have enough choices to please everyone—potatoes, rice, beans, and pasta, to name just a few. And, when we want to take an all-day hike to explore our new planet, we will be able to do what athletes often do before a big race—"carbo-load."

To carbo-load means to load up on starches—one kind of carbohydrate—and build up stored energy in our bodies. We can then use this energy when we have a lot of work to do over a long period of time. So if we want to build a house or climb a mountain on our planet, carbo-loading will come in pretty handy!

Carbo-loading is not something we would want to do every day, because we need to eat a well-balanced diet to remain healthy. But carbo-loading is something that athletes can try if their doctors say it's okay.

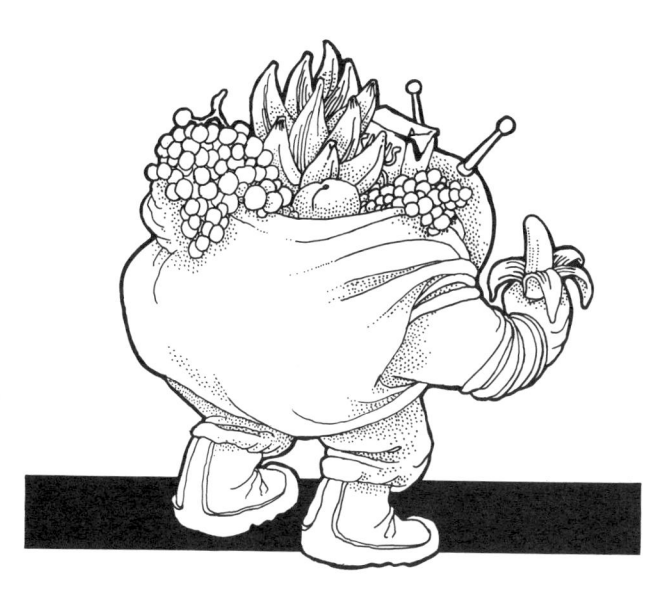

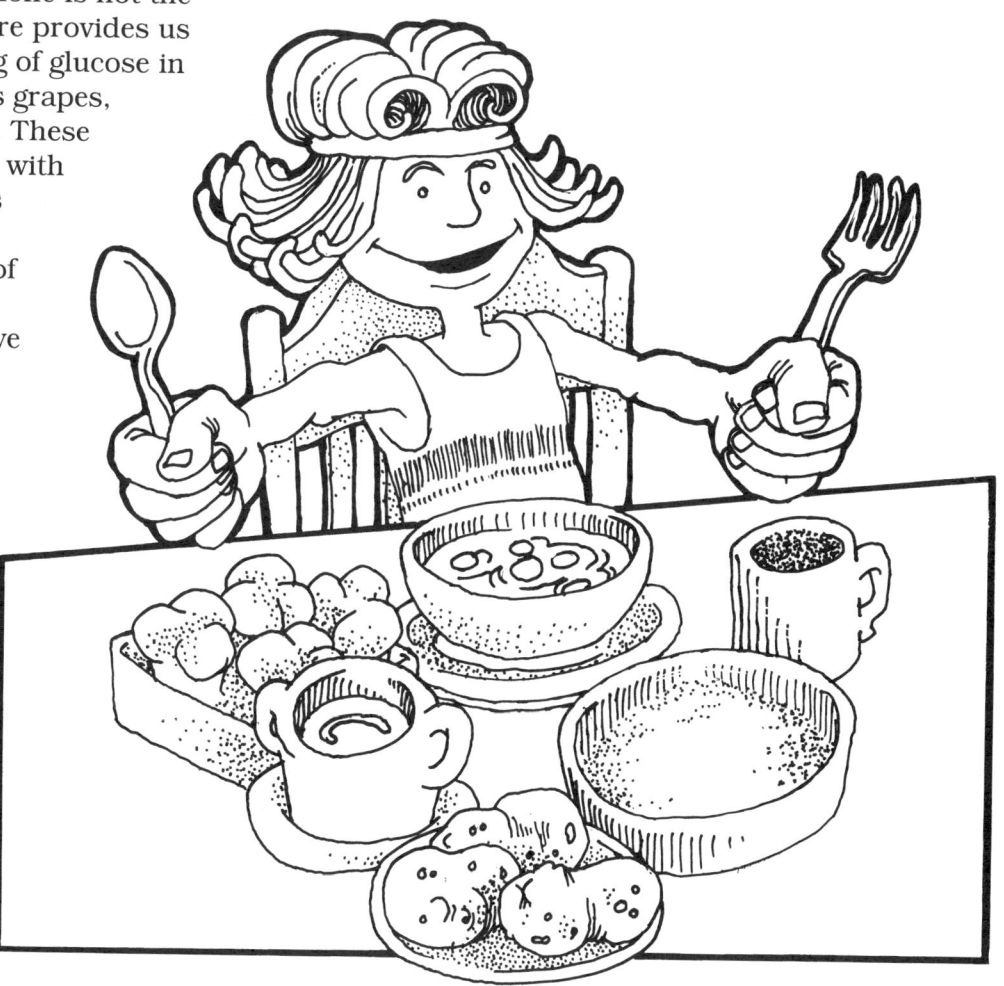

bodies to develop more fat than we need to stay healthy. In fact, being overweight can cause even more problems with our health.

Nature's Sweeteners

If we intend to stay healthy and active on our new planet, glucose alone is not the answer. Luckily, nature provides us with a healthy helping of glucose in certain fruits, such as grapes, raisins, and bananas. These foods also provide us with other useful nutrients our bodies need.

When our ship full of starches does come, we will once again have

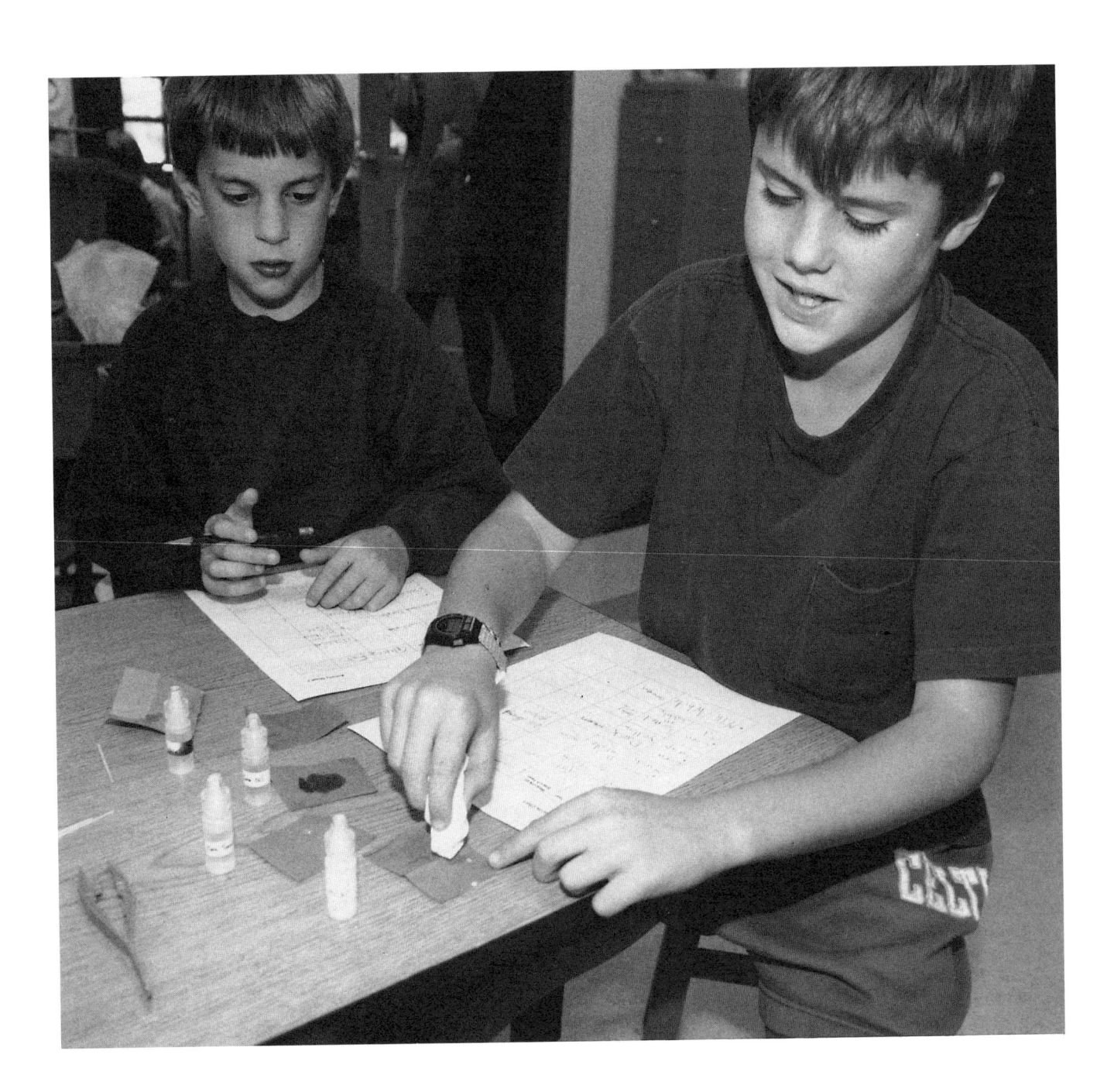

| LESSON 9 | **Testing Liquids for Fats** |

Overview and Objectives

To test for starch, students added iodine to the liquids and foods. And to test for glucose, they used an enzyme-treated test paper. In this lesson, students learn to test for fats by using only unglazed brown paper and discover that some tests are simpler than others. Also, beginning in this lesson, students are challenged to create data tables on their own. As the unit progresses, you can use these individual tables to assess each student's ability to apply the skills he or she has been practicing—collecting, organizing, recording, and analyzing data.

- Each student designs a data table to record results from the fats test.

- Students make predictions and test the liquids for the presence or absence of fats.

- Students record and discuss their findings about the fats test.

- Using their analysis of the test data, students establish a positive and negative test for fats.

- Students research basic facts about fats.

Background

Our bodies need fat to insulate us from the cold, cushion us from bruises and injury, and provide us with energy. Our bodies store fat and use it when other energy sources are unavailable.

It is important to realize that talking about body fat is not the same as talking about fats in foods. Per pound, the fats in food provide twice as much energy as carbohydrates (sugars and starches). In addition, fats come from both animal and plant sources. Nuts, fatty meats, cream, and chocolate are some foods that have a high fat content.

As illustrated in Figure 9-1, there are two kinds of fats—saturated and unsaturated. In general, experts think that diets rich in saturated fats may be related to an increased incidence of heart disease. While various guidelines differ, many experts recommend that less than 30% of the calories in a person's diet be fat.

This lesson's simple test for fats is based on one of the nutrient's physical properties; that is, when foods containing fats are rubbed on certain materials (such as a lunch bag, paper towel, or orange construction paper), the fats leave a grease spot on the paper that does not dry out. Initially, water produces a similar spot; however, unlike the spot left by fats, the water spot evaporates and eventually disappears.

Figure 9-1

How fats are classified

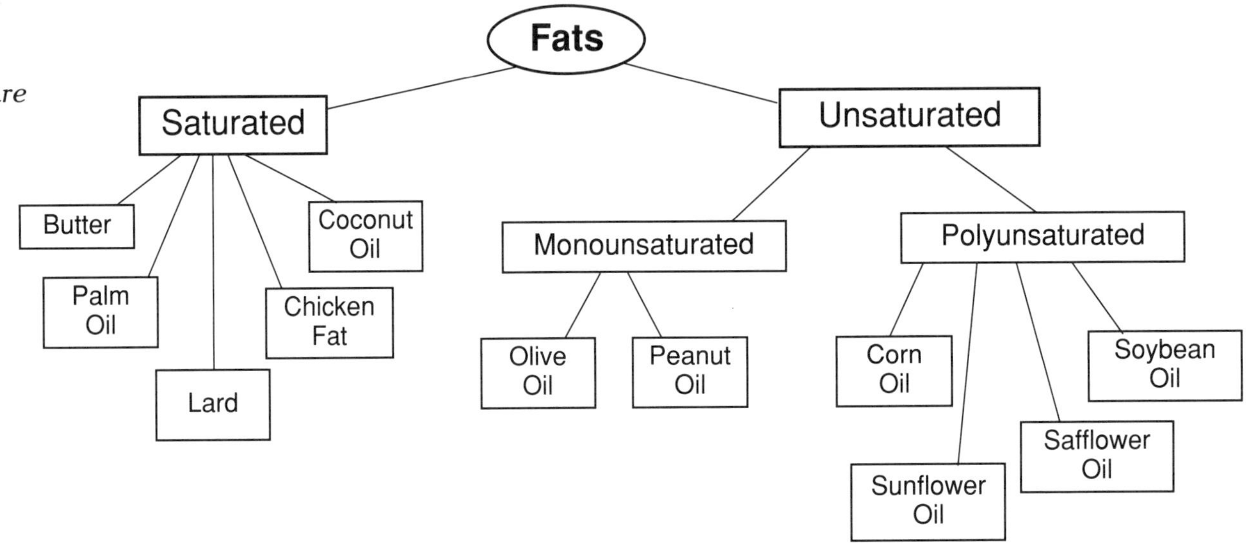

```
                        Fats
                       /    \
                Saturated   Unsaturated
                              /      \
                   Monounsaturated   Polyunsaturated
```

Saturated: Butter, Coconut Oil, Palm Oil, Chicken Fat, Lard

Monounsaturated: Olive Oil, Peanut Oil

Polyunsaturated: Corn Oil, Soybean Oil, Sunflower Oil, Safflower Oil

---

As mentioned in Lesson 1, fats are in almost all foods. However, the amount of fat contained in a food or liquid may affect results when that food is tested. For example, in this test, corn oil is one substance that—due to its high fat content—will yield a clear positive test result. Foods and liquids with lower fat content (such as corn syrup) may produce only a very faint grease spot. Foods with little fat content may leave no grease spot. Students may need guidance when interpreting these results.

Students will learn more about fat and the role it plays in nutrition from reading "Some Good News About Fat," on pg. 116 in Lesson 11. For more in-depth information on fat, you may wish to preview the **Reading Selection** now.

Materials

For each student
1 science notebook

For every four students
1 storage bag containing the following:
  1 food bag
  2 lab bags
  1 liquids bag
2 paper towels
2 brown paper lunch bags
2 rulers
2 pairs of scissors

For the class
1 carton of skim milk, 237 ml (½ pt)
2 clean jars with lids, for mixing 100 ml (3½ oz) quantities of liquid cornstarch and dilute corn syrup
1 measuring spoon, 5 ml (1 tsp)
1 graduated plastic cup, 100 ml (4½ oz)

LESSON 9

1 "Class Liquids Test Table," from Lessons 3 and 6, and large marker
Newsprint or poster board, or overhead transparency and pen
Cleanup materials (2 plastic-lined disposal boxes, sponges, paper towels)
Soapy water (sink or buckets)
Clear water (sink or buckets)

Preparation

1. As you did in Lessons 3 and 6, prepare the cornstarch and corn syrup according to the following directions:

   ■ Cornstarch: Mix together 5 ml (1 tsp) of cornstarch and 100 ml (3½ oz) of tap water.

   ■ Corn syrup: Mix together 5 ml (1 tsp) of corn syrup and 100 ml (3½ oz) of tap water.

2. Have student helpers refill the dropper bottles containing corn syrup, cornstarch, milk, and, if necessary, water and corn oil, and return each set to the liquids bags.

3. Cut a piece of paper approximately 5 cm x 10 cm (2" x 4") from a brown paper bag to use for demonstration purposes.

4. Post the "Class Liquids Test Table."

Management Tip: During the fats test, it will take the paper rectangles about ten minutes to dry before students can observe results. Plan an activity for students to do during that time. One idea is to have them write acrostic poems using the words glucose, starch, carbohydrate, or nutrient (see Figure 9-2).

Procedure

1. Begin by asking students what they know about fats. Record students' ideas on newsprint or an overhead transparency. Or, ask students to record ideas in their notebooks.

2. Follow this discussion with an explanation of how the class will test for fats. Once again, students will start by testing the five liquids to identify positive and negative test results.

3. Explain to students that, starting with this test, they will make their own test tables. Help them recall the tables they used for Lessons 3 and 6 when students were testing liquids for starch and then glucose. Conduct a short discussion based on student ideas about the purpose of these tables and the purpose of each section.

4. Then explain that students can design tables any way they would like, as long as

   ■ The table has an appropriate title and date

   ■ It contains the same information as previous liquids test tables

   ■ The sections are clearly labeled

   ■ The liquids are numbered as they have been

5. Now give students about five to ten minutes to set up their tables. Suggest that they refer to their earlier liquids test tables, if necessary.

6. Next, ask students to talk briefly with their teammates about what they think will happen in the test and then to record their predictions on the new tables.

LESSON 9

Figure 9-2

Sample acrostic poem

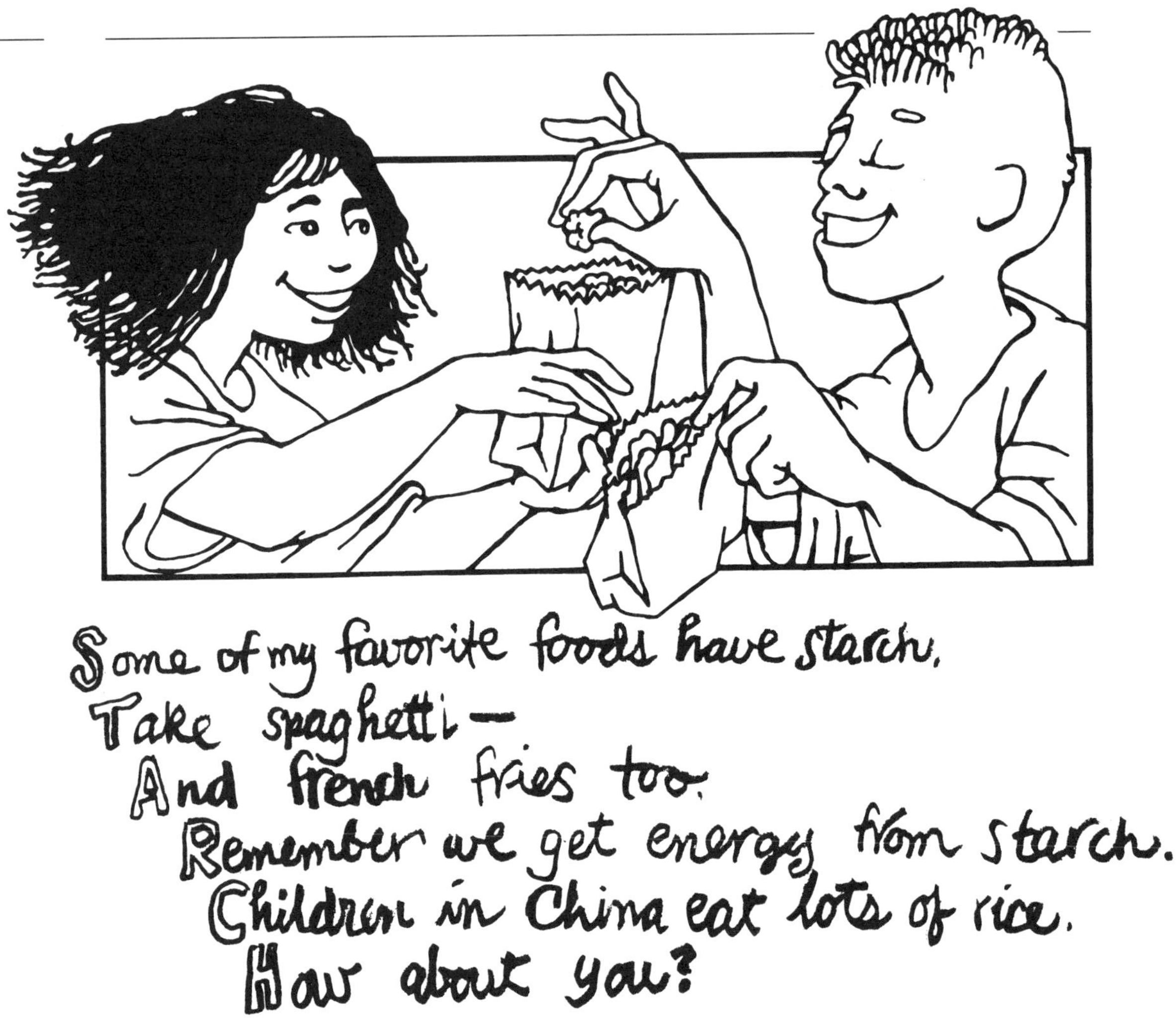

> Some of my favorite foods have starch.
> Take spaghetti —
> And french fries too.
> Remember we get energy from starch.
> Children in China eat lots of rice.
> How about you?

7. Review with students the **Student Instructions for Testing Liquids for Fats** on pg. 45 of the Student Activity book and pg. 103 of this guide.

   Note: Hold up the piece of brown paper you cut earlier and explain that each pair of students will cut 16 pieces—six to use in today's liquids test, and ten to use in the next lesson's foods test.

8. Have one student from each group pick up the following materials and let students begin testing:

   - the group's storage bag
   - 2 paper towels
   - 2 brown paper bags
   - 2 pairs of scissors
   - 2 rulers

9. While the papers dry (it will take about ten minutes), have students work on a related activity (see **Management Tip**, pg. 99).

10. When students have finished discussing and recording their results, have them clean up following the directions below (also found on pg. 44 of the Student Activity Book):

- Put the piece(s) of brown paper that showed a positive result for fats in your notebook to use in Lesson 10. Also put in the unused piece of paper that served as a control.
- Save the other ten unused pieces in your notebook to use in the next lesson.
- Throw away the other paper pieces you used in this test.
- Empty, wash, and rinse out the dropper bottles of cornstarch, corn syrup, and milk. Return all five dropper bottles to your liquids bag and put it back in your storage bag.
- Throw away the used paper towels into the plastic-lined disposal boxes and return all materials to their storage area.

Final Activities

1. Have a member from each group come up to the "Class Liquids Test Table" and write his or her group's test result for each liquid.

2. Then, starting with water, ask the class to describe in detail what happened to the papers when each liquid was added and allowed to dry. Encourage students to discuss the differences between the mark the corn oil made and the marks the other liquids made.

3. Discuss any differing results. Allow time for students to repeat the test later to see if they get the same results.

4. Then have students answer this question in their notebooks:
   - What is the difference between the mark the corn oil made and the marks the other liquids made?

5. Assign each student to find out two facts about fats and be ready to share them in Lesson 10.

Extensions

1. Suggest that students perform the fat test using low-fat milk (1% or 2%), skim milk, whole milk, and cream. Have students make a table to show their results.

2. Encourage students to experiment with other types of paper to test liquids and foods for fat.

3. Ask students what kind of milk they drink at home. Ask them to talk to their parents and find out why.

LESSON 9

Assessments

As students learn to test for a new nutrient, look again for those who demonstrate improved lab procedures and participation in discussion. As you review students' written observations over the next three lessons, look for growth in the following areas.

Student Tables
- Are sections clearly labeled?
- Is all necessary information included?
- Do observations include sufficient detail?

Notebook Entries
- What do students think the word "fat" means? Do they think of fat only in terms of obesity, or do they know it is an important nutrient? Does their perception of fat change by the end of Lesson 11?
- Are students connecting facts from their research and reading to the foods they tested?
- When students compare carbohydrates to fats, do they make distinctions between glucose and starch?

Student Instructions for Testing Liquids for Fats

1. Cut your brown paper lunch bag into 16 rectangles that are about 5 cm x 10 cm (2" x 4") each. Put ten of them back in your notebook to use in Lesson 10.

2. Number the rectangles from one to five to match the numbers and liquids on your liquids table for the fats test. The unnumbered one is the control.

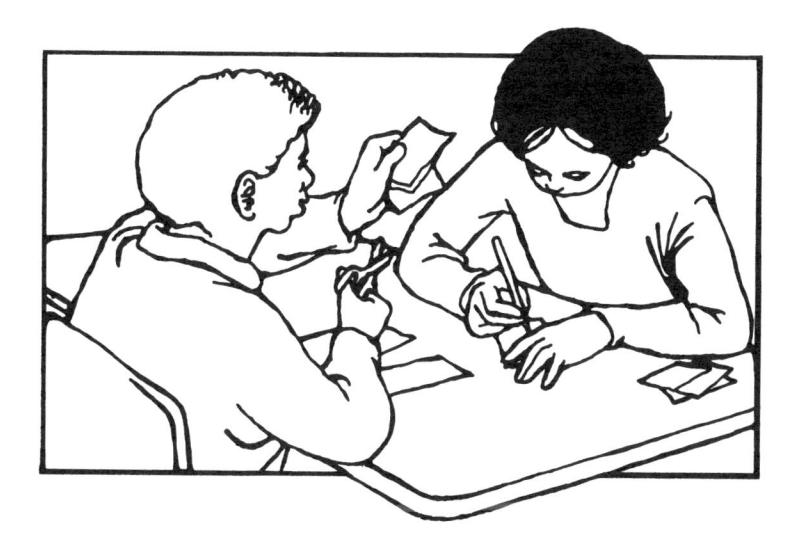

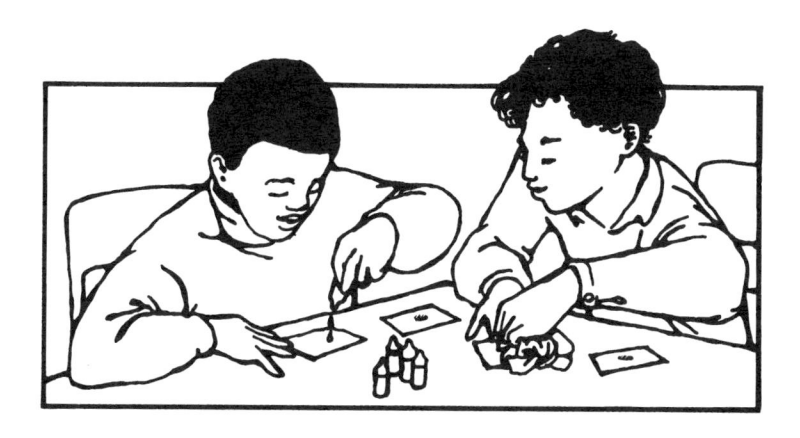

3. On the papers with the corresponding numbers, put two drops of each liquid: water, cornstarch, corn syrup, corn oil, and milk.

4. Use a paper towel to blot the extra liquid from the brown paper.

5. Let the papers dry for about ten minutes.

6. When ten minutes are up, observe the results for each liquid.

STC / *Food Chemistry*

LESSON 9

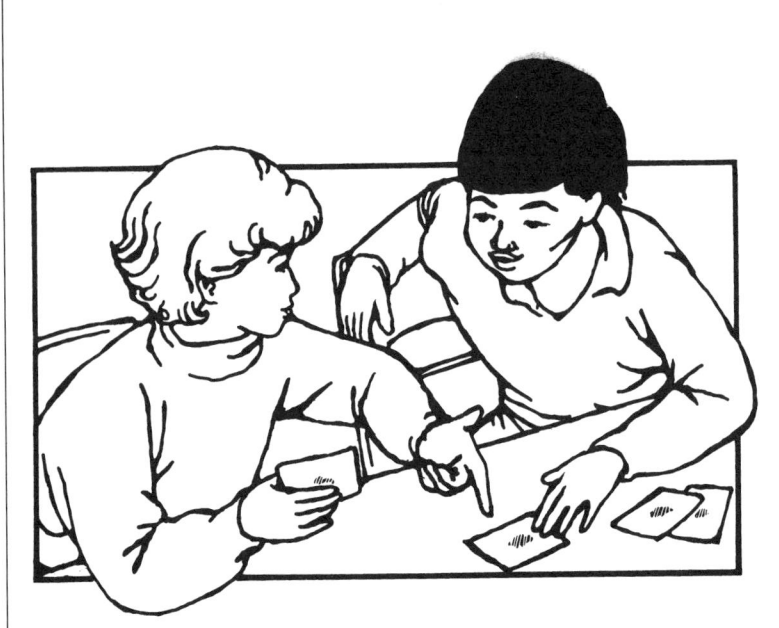

7. Discuss the results with your group and record them on your liquids table for the fats test. Be as descriptive as you can.

8. With your group, decide which liquid(s) tested positive (+) for fats and which tested negative (–). Save any brown test paper with a positive test result on it in your notebook. When you test the foods for fats, you will use the paper(s) and your liquids table from the fats test to compare results.

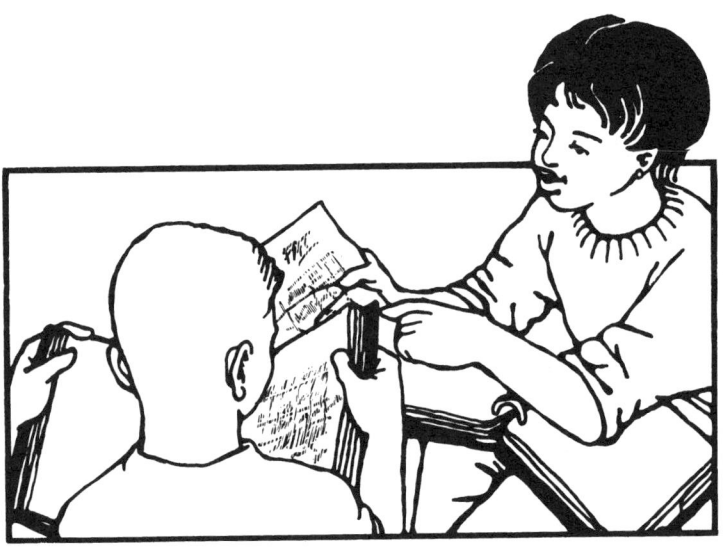

9. Now follow your cleanup instructions.

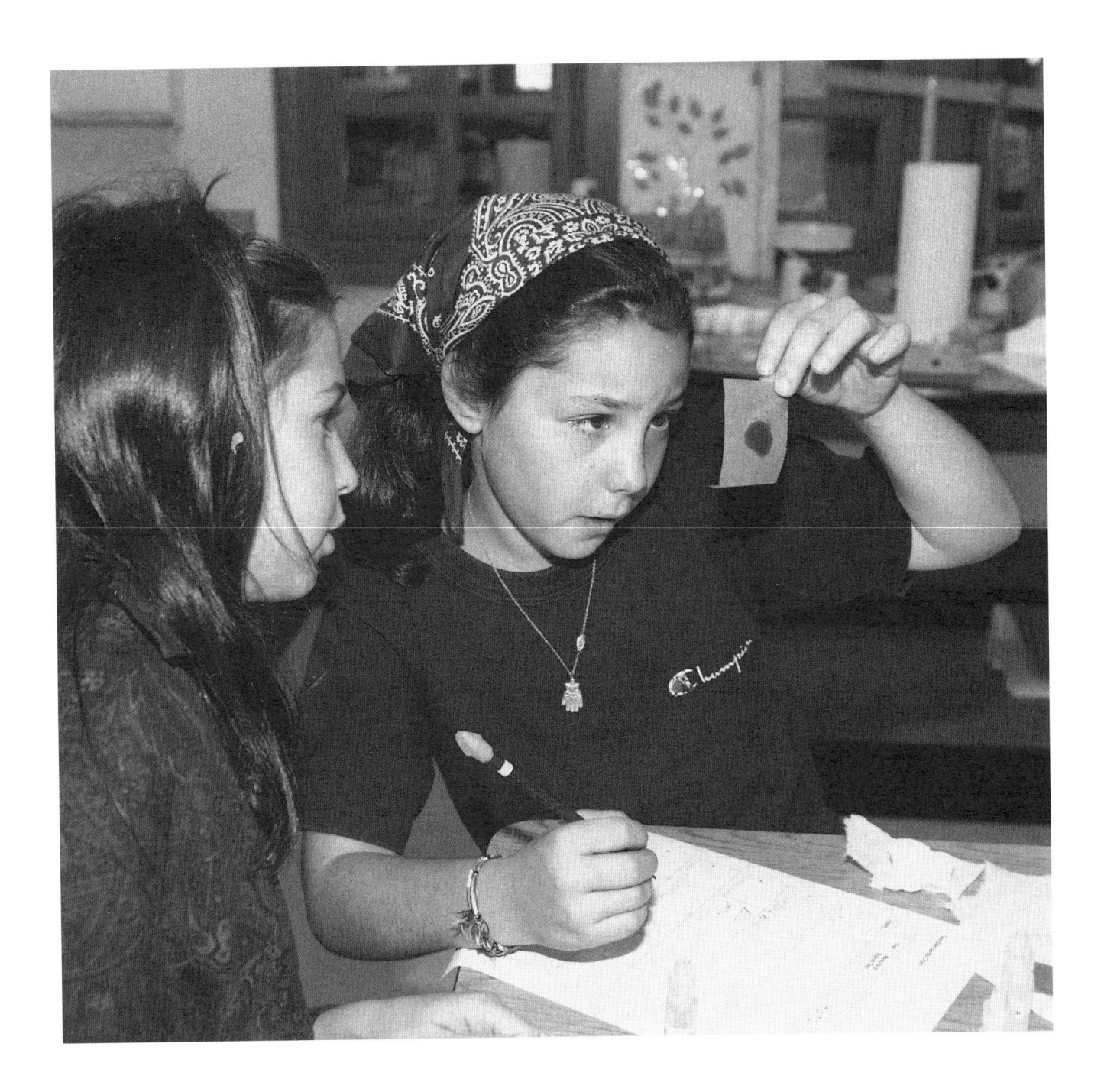

| LESSON 10 | **Testing Foods for Fats** |

Overview and Objectives

Using the simple test learned in Lesson 9, students identify which of their foods contain fats. The class will discover that when fat content varies from food to food, test results can be less conclusive and more open to interpretation. Once again, students apply what they have learned about test tables to design and complete food test tables of their own.

- Students share what they have learned about fats through individual research.

- Students design a data table to record their results for testing foods for fats.

- Students make and record predictions of the foods they think do and do not contain fats.

- Students apply the fats test to their foods, record and analyze results, and compare the range of results with their predictions.

- Students record in their notebooks their observations, discoveries, and questions about fats and the test for fats, and then share these in a class discussion.

Background

A number of factors, including differences in texture, water content, and state (whether the food is solid or liquid) will affect how well the fats test in this lesson works. In general, however, you can expect students' findings to match those shown in Figure 10-1.

Figure 10-1

Results of the Fats Test

Positive	Negative
Peanuts	Rice
Coconut flakes	Egg white
Granola bar	Flour
	Onion
	Apple

LESSON 10

When testing solid foods for fats, students must place each food on each square of paper and rub the food against it, hard. This squeezes out the oils for the paper to absorb.

In earlier tests, students made an effort to avoid contamination by not touching the glucose test papers. But in this test, they must use their fingers to hold the foods and rub them into the paper. Since all humans have natural oil on their fingers, students need to wipe their fingers with a paper towel before touching each test food.

Materials

For each student
1   science notebook, including the individual liquids table for the fats test, from Lesson 9

For every two students
10   pieces of brown paper saved from Lesson 9

For every four students
1   storage bag containing the following:
   1   food bag
   2   lab bags
   1   liquids bag
4   paper towels

For the class
"Class Foods Test Table," from previous lessons, and large marker
Cleanup materials (2 plastic-lined disposal boxes)

Preparation

Display the "Class Foods Test Table."

Procedure

1. Ask students to share the information they discovered about fats. You may also want students to record their facts on a class list.

2. Then ask students how they can use what they learned in Lesson 9 to test their foods for fat.

3. Have students create their own foods test tables. Remind them to include headings and space for all the information collected on the foods test tables for glucose and starch.

4. Now ask students to predict for each food whether or not fat is present and to write the predictions on their tables.

5. Ask some students to volunteer to discuss the reasoning behind their predictions. On what basis did they predict that these foods contain fat?

6. Briefly review the **Student Instructions for Testing Foods for Fats** on pg. 110 in this guide and pg. 49 of the Student Activity Book.

7. Then ask one student from each group to pick up the group's storage bag and let the class start testing.

   Note: When students have finished testing, make sure they put the squares of paper in a safe place to dry and do not accidentally throw them out.

8. During the ten minutes the papers are drying, have students follow the cleanup instructions below (also found on pg. 48 of the Student Activity Book):

- Put the correct lids securely back on the food cups.
- Discard the foods tested—but not the test papers—in the plastic-lined disposal boxes.
- Wipe the spoons with a paper towel and return the food cups and spoons to the food bag.
- Put the food bag back in the storage bag and return it to the storage area.

9. Ask a student from each group to record the group's results on the "Class Foods Test Table."

Final Activities

1. Ask students to write a few sentences in their notebooks answering the following questions:

   - How did today's results compare with the test result for corn oil in terms of size and darkness?
   - How did the results compare with each other in terms of size and darkness?
   - What do you think these differences indicate about the amount of fat in each food?
   - Which foods contain starch, glucose, and fat? Which contain starch and fat but not glucose?
   - What questions do you have about fats and the test for fats?

2. When they are finished, ask students to share their answers in a class discussion.

Extensions

1. Have students test a variety of cooking oils for fat. Are the results the same for each?

2. Have the class write letters to companies that produce "low-fat" products, such as milk, yogurt, and salad dressing, and ask how each company's low-fat and high-fat products differ.

3. Invite a guest chef to talk to the class about different cooking fats and how chefs use them.

4. Ask students to find out what kind of materials are used to wrap or contain fatty foods such as candy bars, butter, french fries, and ice cream. Then discuss what students think about why these materials are used.

LESSON 10

Student Instructions for Testing Foods for Fats

1. Remove the ten pieces of brown paper from your notebook and number them from one to ten.

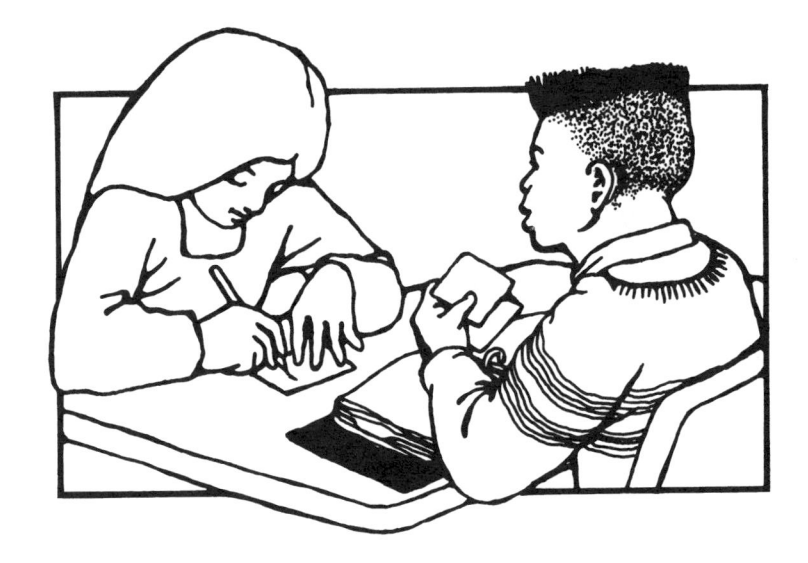

2. In this test, the peanut is the only food that needs special preparation. Remove the peanut's shell and papery coating.

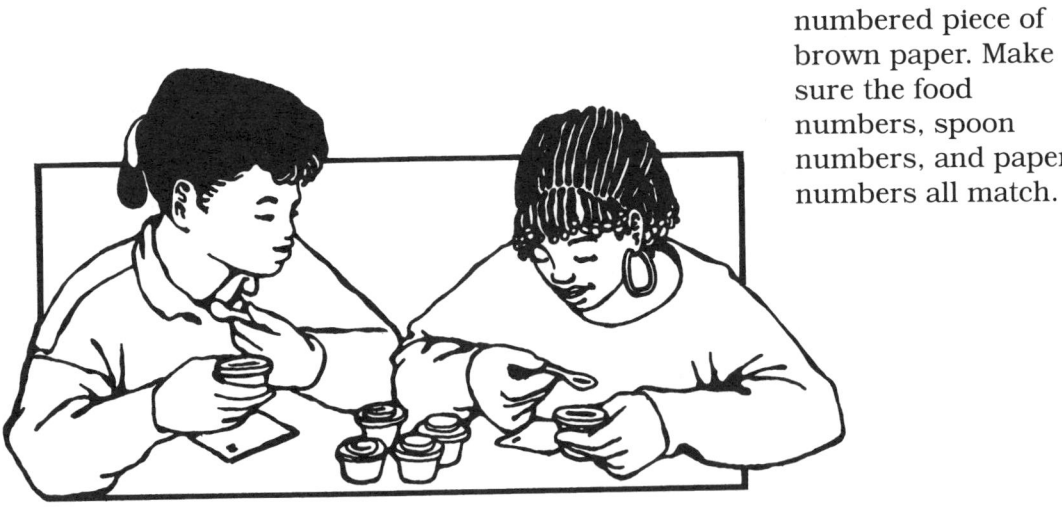

3. For this simple test, you do not need your test tray. Instead, put one small spoon of each food on a numbered piece of brown paper. Make sure the food numbers, spoon numbers, and paper numbers all match.

LESSON 10

4. Wipe your fingers with a paper towel. Then, with your fingers, take food No. 1 (rice) and rub it hard against paper No. 1.

5. Repeat this process for the other foods. **Be sure to wipe your fingers** after you test each food and before you test the next one.

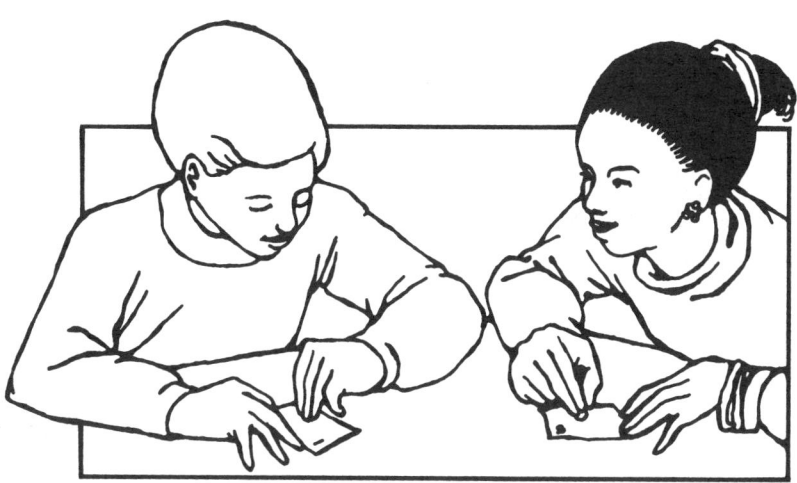

6. After you have tested all the foods, put the papers in a safe place and let them dry for about ten minutes.

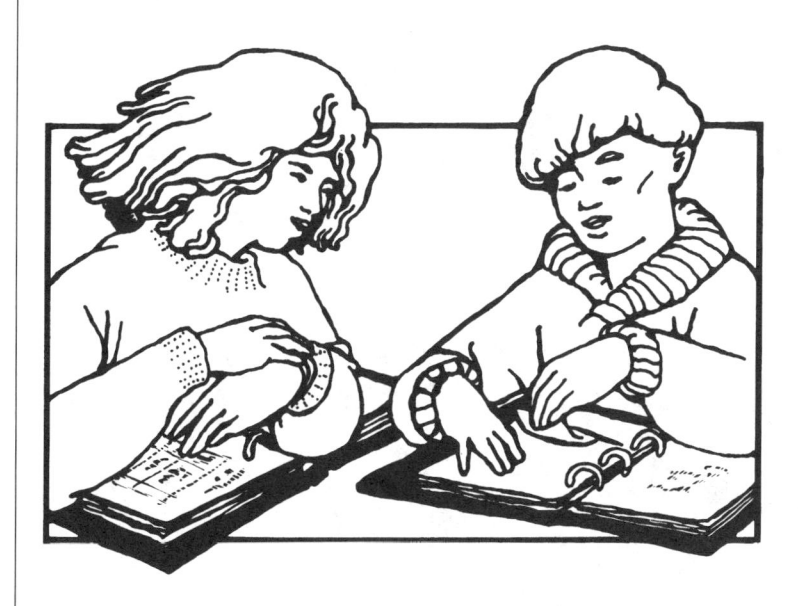

7. While the papers are drying, clean up. **Do not throw out the test papers!**

8. Take out the paper that showed a positive test during the liquids testing. After ten minutes, observe the reaction for each food and compare the papers to this positive test paper. Also look at the results on your liquids table for the fats test.

9. Record observations on your foods table for the fats test. Be as descriptive as you can.

10. Follow your cleanup instructions.

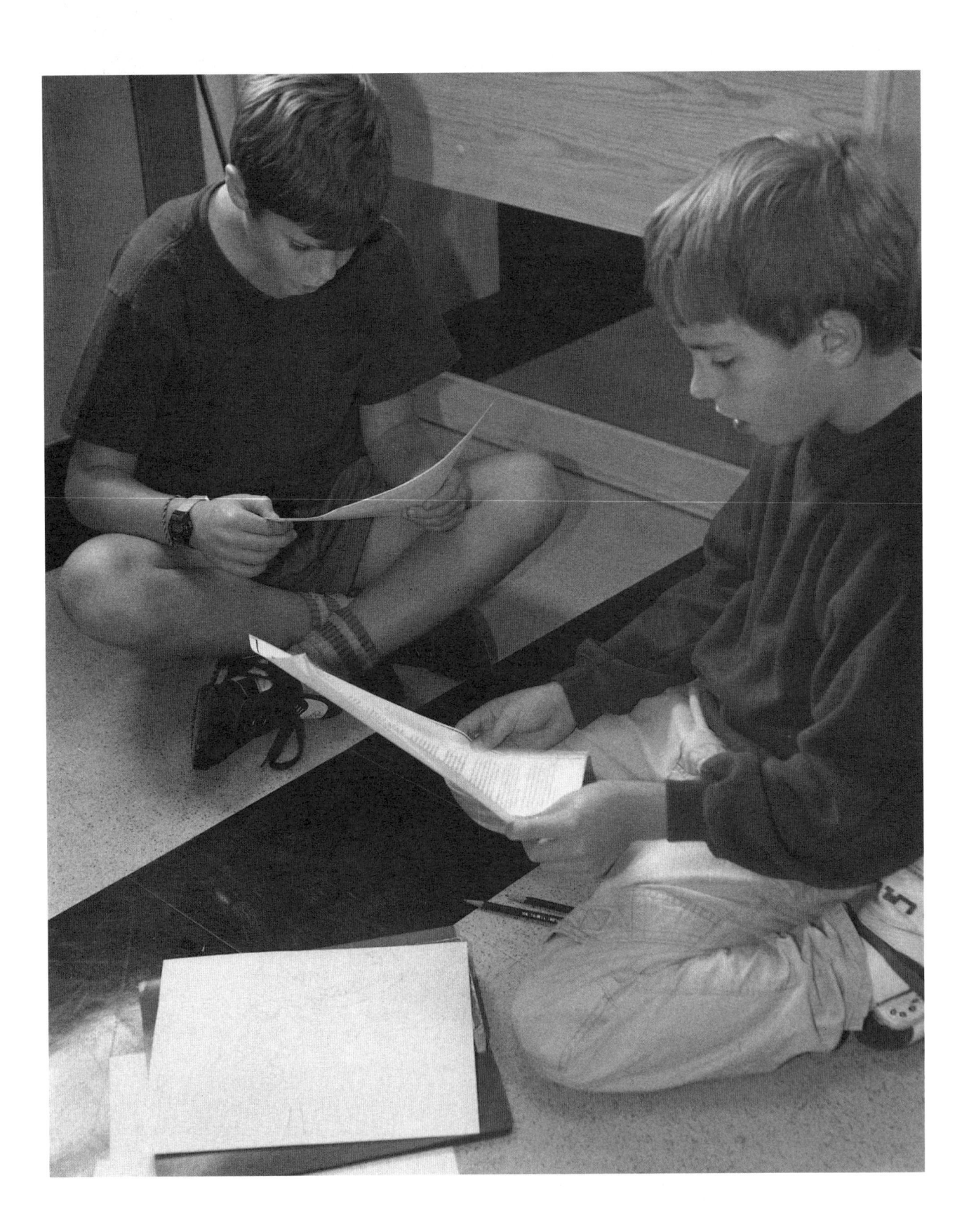

LESSON 11

Learning More about Fats

Overview and Objectives

This lesson provides another opportunity for students to consider why test results may differ, to validate results through retesting, and to observe and discuss the range of positive results. Through readings and discussions, students also begin to discover that fat, in addition to being an aspect of their body weight, plays an important role in their health.

- Students analyze their results from testing their foods for fat and discuss why different results may have occurred.
- The class retests foods for which results vary.
- Students read and write about the role fats play in their diets.
- Through class discussion and writing, students compare fats with carbohydrates.

Background

Our understanding of health and diet is changing as we learn more about human nutrition and the roles various foods play. As students explore issues about fat, let them know that the scientific community still has many questions about the human diet and which foods are good for us and which are not. Encourage students to think about the fact that these questions do not have simple answers and that, as scientists continue to conduct research on human nutrition, new and important information will emerge.

Materials

For each student
  1   science notebook, including the individual foods test table for the fats test, from Lesson 10

For every four students (for retesting, if needed)
  1   storage bag containing the following:
     1   food bag
     2   lab bags
     1   liquids bag
  2   brown paper bags
  2   pairs of scissors
  2   rulers
  2   paper towels

LESSON 11

For the class
> "Class Foods Test Table," from previous lessons
> "Questions We Have about Foods" list, from previous lessons, and large marker

Preparation

1. Post the "Class Foods Test Table." Make sure the "Questions We Have about Foods" list is still posted.

2. Read "Some Good News about Fat," on pg. 116.

Procedure

1. Ask students to share what they have learned about the amount of fat in their test foods. In the discussion, they should refer to their notebooks, especially to their individual foods test tables from Lesson 10.

2. Also have the class look at the "Class Foods Test Table" for each group's fats test results and discuss how the results compare.

3. If students have obtained different results, ask them to think back to earlier tests in which results differed and the reasons why this may have happened. After students retest and record their data, have them discuss the new results.

Management Tip: If retesting and discussing second test results take too much time, you may want to have students do the rest of the lesson, beginning with the **Reading Selection**, as homework or during language arts.

4. Now ask students to read "Some Good News about Fat," (on pg. 53 in their Student Activity Books and pg. 116 of this guide).

Final Activities

1. When students have finished reading, ask them to review their notes, tables, record sheets, and reading selections for information that will help them to compare carbohydrates with fats. Then have students write several comparisons in their notebooks. To get the class started, briefly discuss the following questions:

   - What is meant by fat?
   - What are some foods that contain fats?
   - What are some foods that contain both carbohydrates and fats?
   - How are carbohydrates and fats alike?
   - How are carbohydrates and fats different?

2. Have students add any new questions they may have to the "Questions We Have about Foods" list.

Extensions

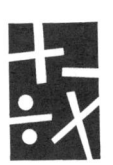

1. Ask students to bring in packages of snack foods they like. Hold up each food and ask students to raise their hands if they like it. Then, have students find the fat content on each food's label. The class can report the survey results on a scatterplot (see Figure 11-1), as a means of illustrating correlations between each snack and its fat content. When students make the scatterplot, suggest that they use different shapes or different colored dots to represent the different categories of foods.

114 / Learning More about Fats

Figure 11-1

Sample scatterplot

CORRELATION OF FAT CONTENT TO PREFERRED FOODS

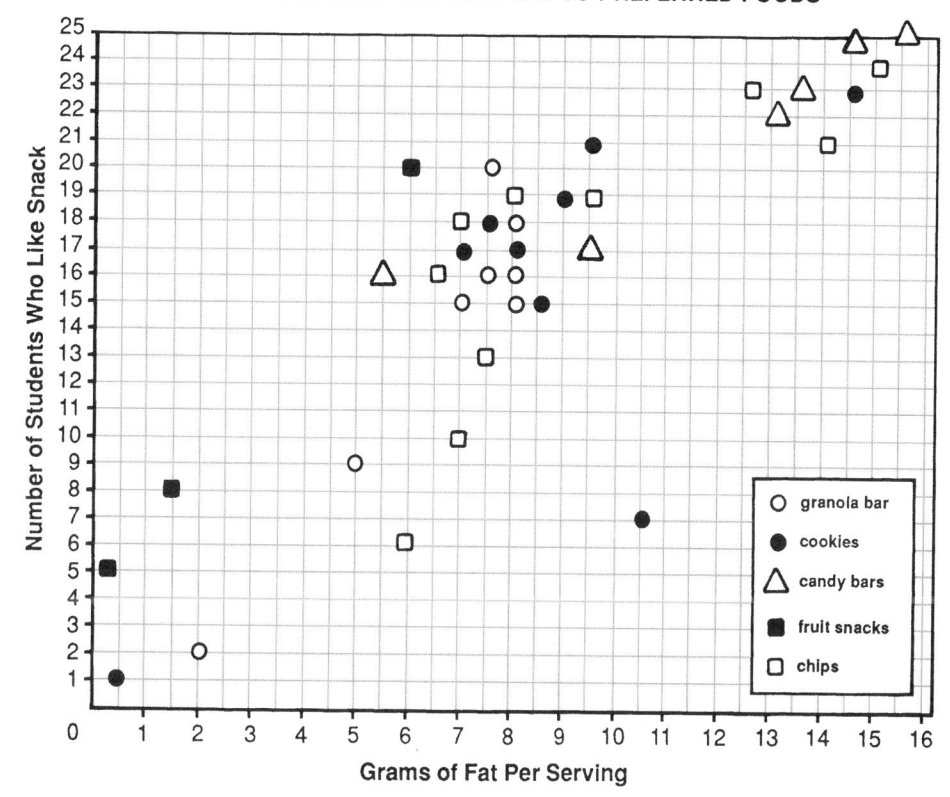

[Scatterplot: x-axis "Grams of Fat Per Serving" (0–16), y-axis "Number of Students Who Like Snack" (0–25). Legend: ○ granola bar, ● cookies, △ candy bars, ■ fruit snacks, □ chips.]

On this scatterplot, each symbol represents a different type of snack food (potato chips, granola bars, candy bars, and so forth). In this sample, most students liked foods with a fat content of about 7-8 grams. If your class does this on a large class grid, they may want to use colored dots to represent the different foods.

2. Invite students to find articles about fats and other nutrients and bring them into class. Create (and continue to add to) a "nutrient" bulletin board to spark future class discussions or student news reports.

3. Challenge students to role-play a nutrient or a specific food and give a short speech telling about themselves.

4. Encourage students to test cafeteria foods for fats.

Assessments

To help you assess student growth at this time, you may want to refer back to the **Assessments** section on pg. 102 of Lesson 9.

Reading Selection

Some Good News about Fat

Have you heard the good news about fat? Gram per gram, fat is just about the most energy-packed source of food for your body. The bad news about fat is that it's easy to get too much of it. And too much fat can be bad for your health.

A gram of fat contains more than two times as much energy as a gram of carbohydrate (starch and glucose) or protein. Fat causes you to feel full after you eat it. It also helps protect your bones and cushion your organs. And, the fat tissue in your body stores some of the vitamins you need.

If you were an explorer trudging through the Arctic wilderness, you'd choose a diet with lots of fat in it—for example, one with nuts, fatty meats, and chocolate. Remember, fat gives you a lot of energy for its weight. So you could lighten your backpack by carrying less food.

Also, these foods would help to keep you warm. How? Your body stores the fat it doesn't use for energy. That fat works like an extra sweater to insulate you from the cold.

On the other hand, if you worked in an office and spent most of the day sitting at a desk, you probably would cut down on your fatty foods. You wouldn't need the extra energy, and your body would most likely just store the fat rather than use it.

Some fatty foods have a bad reputation, and for valid reasons. Still, you don't want to stop eating fat completely. A healthy diet should include fat, but the amount should vary based on factors such as your age, total weight, and individual needs.

All Fats Are Not Equal

When are fats considered "bad"? When they cause health problems. Saturated fats are the fats which cause concern for many people. Saturated fats are found in both plants and animals, but primarily in animals.

So, think about this for a moment. Do you eat a bunch of foods fried in animal fats like lard or butter? Do you frequently eat eggs, cheese, or ice cream? These contain saturated fats. And saturated fats may raise the level of cholesterol in your blood.

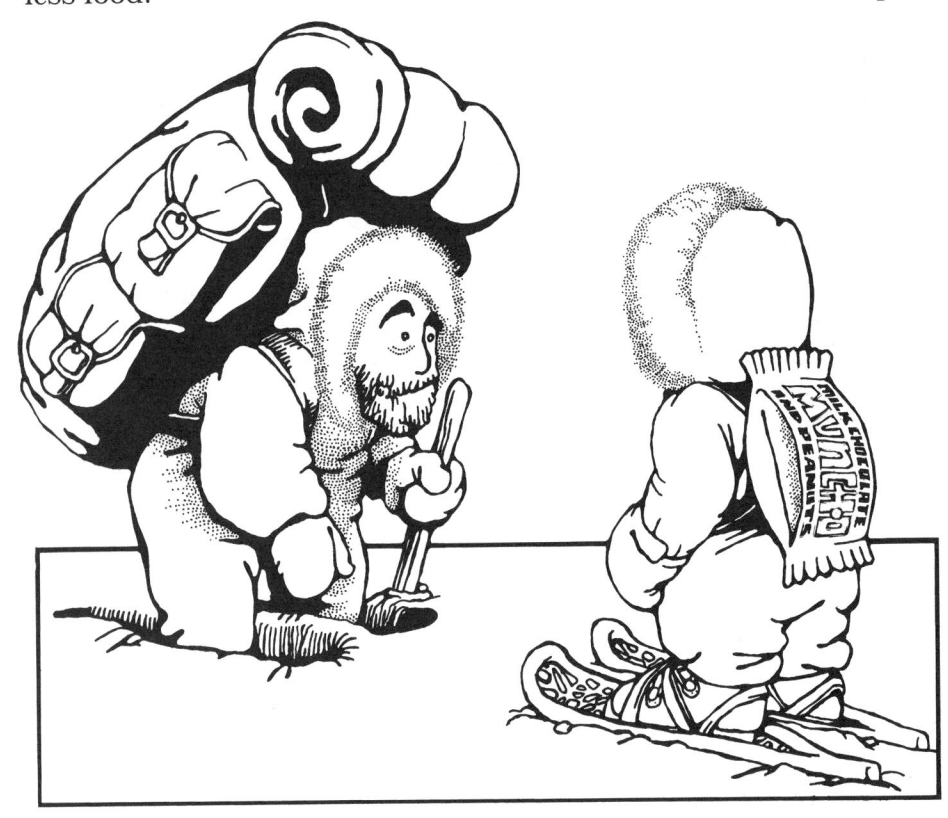

Cholesterol is a soft, fat-like substance found in all your body's cells. It's an important part of a healthy body, and your liver actually makes some cholesterol on its own. But if the saturated fats you eat add to the body's production of cholesterol, it can build up in your arteries. This causes your heart to work too hard to pump your blood. Over time, it can increase the risk of heart disease.

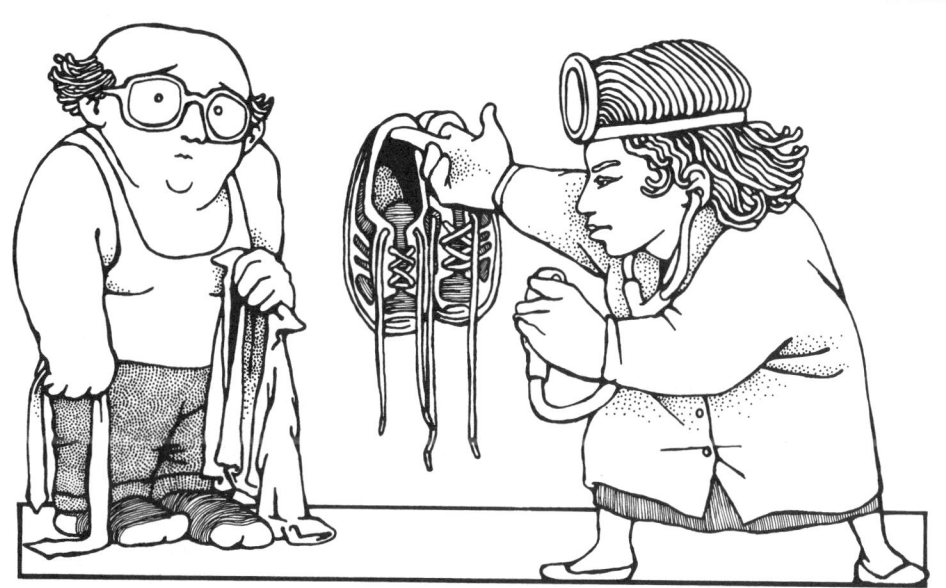

Keep in mind that high cholesterol affects some people more than others. As you grow older, your doctor may suggest that you exercise regularly, cut down on high-fat foods, and have your level of cholesterol and triglycerides (fat) in your blood checked.

Unsaturated fats include cooking oils from seeds, nuts, and vegetables. They usually remain liquid at room temperature. And a number of nutritionists believe that unsaturated fats give your body the "good" fat it needs.

Today, it may seem like any amount of fat is bad. At the supermarket, shoppers reach for foods that are nonfat, or 98% fat-free. And we constantly see advertisements telling us we need to diet. But the simple fact is that a small amount of fat is necessary in the diet. You just shouldn't overdo it. And when you do eat fat, you should try to eat more of the unsaturated kind.

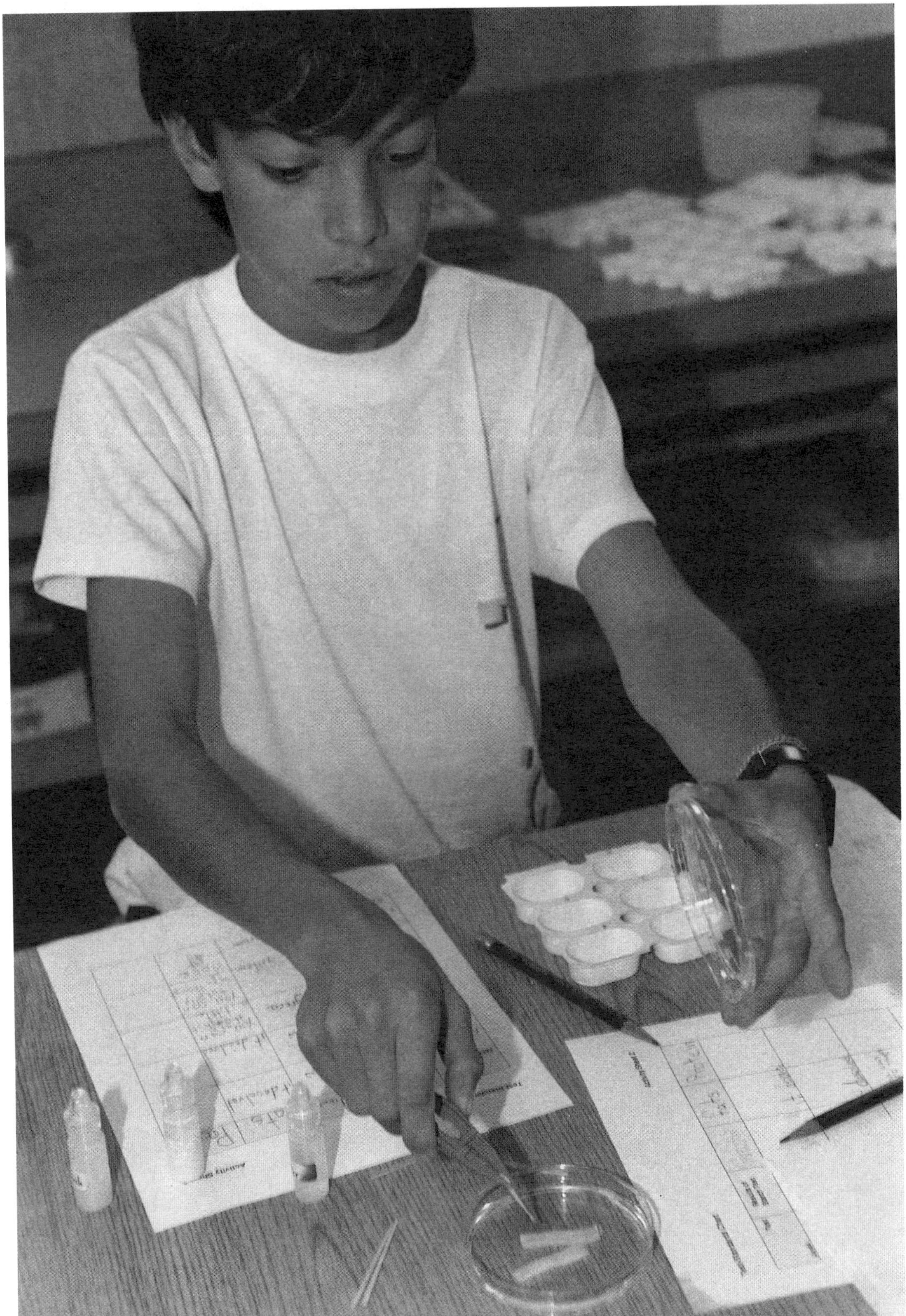

LESSON 12

Testing Liquids for Proteins

Overview and Objectives

Protein is the last nutrient students will study in this unit. Unlike previous tests, the proteins test introduces students to the concept that color changes in the test paper indicate the absence—rather than the presence—of the nutrient for which they are testing. This more complex test also produces a wider and less conclusive range of results. Also in this lesson, students use their cumulative data from the starch, glucose, fats, and proteins tests to discover that water does not contain any of the food nutrients they have studied.

- Students make predictions, test liquids for the presence or absence of protein, and record results on data tables they have designed.

- Students analyze the data they collect to establish a positive and negative test for protein.

- Students record and discuss their findings about the test for protein.

- Students research basic facts about proteins.

Background

Proteins are found in all living things, including both plants and animals. As a source of amino acids (the substances our bodies need to build and repair tissue), proteins are essential to human life. Our digestive system breaks proteins apart into the amino acids we need.

Eggs, cheese, meat, fish, and legumes are some foods that contain large proportions of proteins; however, animal sources generally contain proteins in greater concentrations than plant sources do. Many plants make "incomplete" proteins; that is, they do not contain the full range of amino acids needed for human metabolism. Animal proteins are complete.

But we should not depend on eating only animal proteins and no plant proteins. For one thing, some animal proteins are found in foods that also have a high fat content. For another, animal proteins can be expensive and, in many parts of the world, difficult to obtain. Whatever forms of protein we choose, approximately 120 grams (4 ounces) of protein per day will more than satisfy our bodies' needs.

In today's test, the chemical test material is Coomassie blue paper, also called protein test paper. This test differs from earlier ones in two ways:

- After students immerse the test paper in the liquid or the food, they must develop it in a solution for several minutes.

LESSON 12

- In a positive test, the test paper does not change from one color to another. Instead, the original color of the paper remains. What is also important is the amount of color that is present. Figure 12-1 illustrates how to interpret different results for the protein test.

Figure 12-1

How to Interpret Protein Test Results

Results	What the Result Means
Blue color remains	Liquid or food contains protein
Blue color fades	Liquid or food contains small amount of protein
Blue color almost disappears	Liquid or food contains no protein

The results shown occur because the chemical Coomassie blue actually binds to protein. And because of this chemical reaction, the protein and Coomassie blue will remain on the test paper after students dip it into the developing solution. Conversely, in the absence of protein, the Coomassie blue will dissolve after students dip the paper into the developing solution, causing the color to disappear.

In this test, milk is the only liquid that will have a positive test result for protein, and the test paper used for it will be the only one on which the blue color will remain.

Although water has tested negative for the nutrients students studied in this unit—starch, glucose, fats, and proteins—water is essential to our health. In fact, as mentioned in Lesson 1, it too is a macronutrient. Students may have difficulty grasping the fact that water is a nutrient, but it is important to have them discuss that we cannot live without water and that our bodies need it in large amounts.

Note: Students will learn more about proteins and the role they play in nutrition from reading "Proteins: The Building Blocks of Life," on pg. 140 in Lesson 14. For more in-depth information on proteins, you may wish to preview the **Reading Selection** at this time.

Materials

For each student
  1   science notebook

For every four students
  1   storage bag containing the following:
      1   food bag
      2   lab bags
      1   liquids bag
  2   petri dishes
  1   envelope of 34 strips of Coomassie blue test paper (protein test paper)

LESSON 12

Note: Directions for making your own protein test papers are provided in **Appendix C** on pg. 179.

4 paper towels

For the class
- 1 "Class Liquids Test Table," from previous lessons, and large marker
- 5 funnels
- 2 clean jars with lids, for mixing 100 ml (3½ oz) quantities of liquid cornstarch and dilute corn syrup
- 1 carton of skim milk, 237 ml (½ pt)
- 1 bottle of white vinegar, .5 liter (1 pt)
- 1 bottle of rubbing alcohol, .5 liter (1 pt)
- 1 plastic bottle to mix and store developing solution, 1 liter (1 qt)
- 5 notecards, 12.5 cm x 20 cm (5" x 8"), on which to mount class results
- 1 roll of clear plastic tape

    Newsprint or poster board, or overhead transparency and pen
    Paper towels
    Cleanup materials (2 plastic-lined disposal boxes, sponges, paper towels)
    Soapy water (sink or buckets)
    Clear water (sink or buckets)

Preparation

1. As you did in Lessons 3, 6, and 9, prepare the cornstarch and corn syrup.
    - Cornstarch: Mix together 5 ml (1 tsp) of cornstarch and 100 ml (3½ oz) of tap water.
    - Corn syrup: Mix together 5 ml (1 tsp) of corn syrup and 100 ml (3½ oz) of tap water.

2. Have student helpers refill the dropper bottles containing water, corn syrup, cornstarch, and milk and return each set to the liquids bags.

3. Post the "Class Liquids Test Table."

4. You will need to prepare about 1 liter (1 qt) of developing solution for the protein test papers.
    - Mix together .5 liter (1 pt) of white vinegar with .5 liter (1 pt) of rubbing alcohol in the plastic quart mixing bottle. Store the solution in the closed bottle.

5. Ask student helpers to use forceps to put 34 strips of protein test paper into an envelope for each group of four students. Tell students to be careful not to touch the blue end of each paper.

Note: Each pair of students will use six strips today and the other eleven strips when they test the foods for protein in Lesson 13. In the foods test, students will use a new control strip rather than the one used for the liquids test, since the first control strip will have become contaminated from the developing solution.

LESSON 12

Procedure

1. Begin by asking students what nutrients they have tested for so far. Then ask what they know about proteins. Record students' ideas on newsprint or an overhead transparency. Or, ask students to record ideas quickly in their notebooks.

2. Explain that, today, the class will test for proteins, and that, once again, students will design their own tables to record test results. Hold a brief class discussion to review the necessary elements of a useful table and let students know that the chemical test material is protein test paper. Then have students make their tables.

3. Next, ask students to talk briefly with their groups about which liquids they think will test positive for protein and which they think will test negative. Have students record these predictions on their tables.

4. Hold up a strip of the protein test paper. Explain that, like the glucose test paper, this paper has a special chemical on it—called Coomassie blue—that reacts with protein. Then explain that when a liquid or food being tested contains protein, this test paper will stay blue. But when the liquid or food contains little or no protein, the blue will fade or disappear. Help them understand that the depth of blue color remaining on the paper corresponds to the amount of protein in the food.

5. Review the **Student Instructions for Testing Liquids for Proteins** on pg. 126 of this guide and on pg. 59 of the Student Activity Book. Remind students that touching the blue end of the test papers with their fingers may contaminate results, so they need to use forceps and keep the forceps only on the white end of each strip.

6. Ask one student from each group of four to pick up the following:
   - the group's storage bag
   - 1 envelope containing 34 strips of protein test paper
   - 2 petri dishes

7. Then let the class get to work. As students begin the test, pour into each dish just enough developing solution to cover the bottom completely (see Figure 12-2) but no more than about .5 cm (¼") deep. Keep these dishes covered to control the sharp odor of vinegar.

8. While the papers are developing, ask students to write in their notebooks two questions they would like to answer about proteins. They will later research answers to these questions.

9. After the papers are developed, ask students to discuss results with their group and then to record them on their own test tables.

10. Now choose five student helpers to make displays of the protein test papers while the rest of the class cleans up.
    - Give each helper a notecard.
    - Assign a different liquid to each helper and have him or her label the notecard with the name of that liquid.
    - Have the helpers collect all the protein test papers for that liquid and then tape them onto the card (see Figure 12-3).
    - Display the mounted test results in the classroom.

Figure 12-2

Distributing developing solution

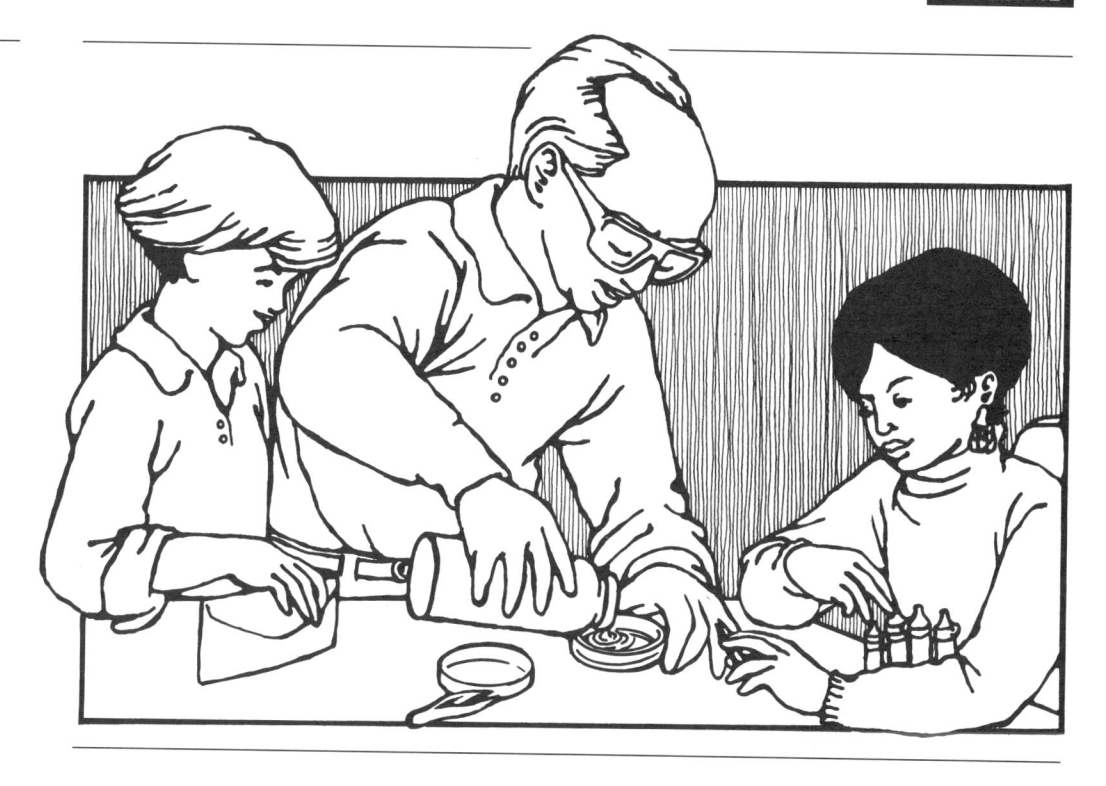

Figure 12-3

Mounted test results

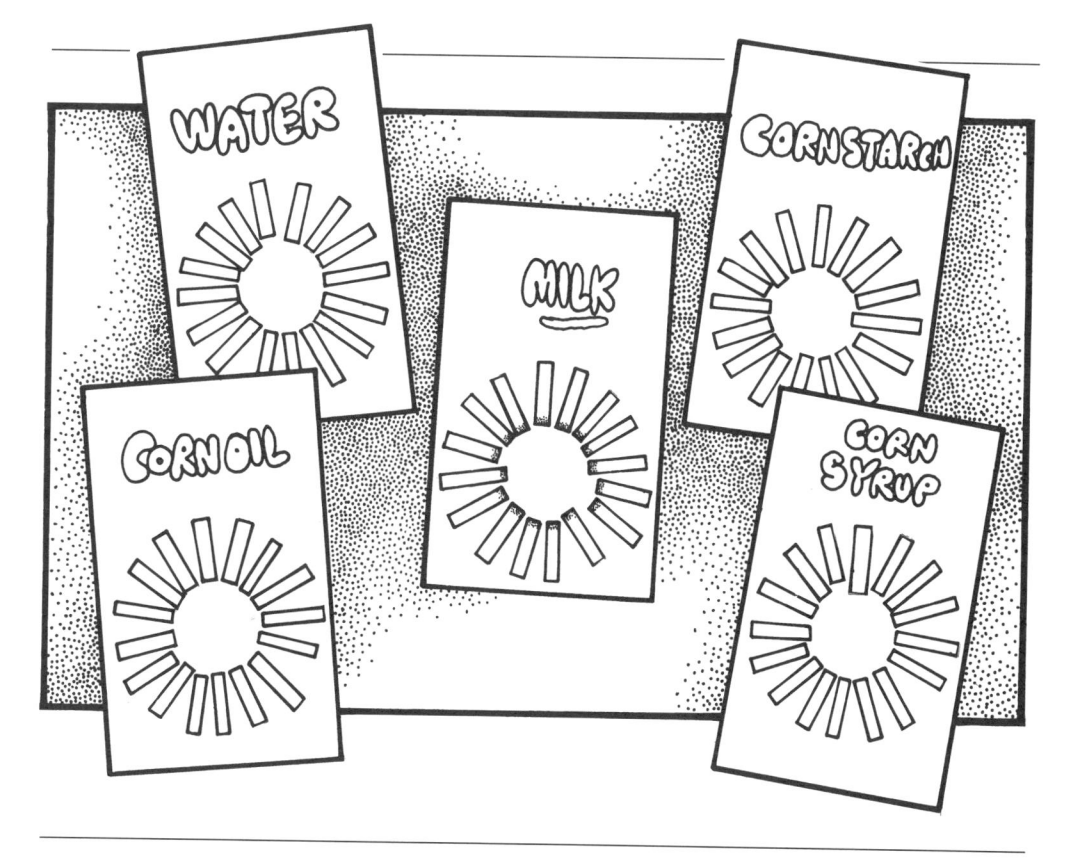

STC / *Food Chemistry* Testing Liquids for Proteins / **123**

LESSON 12

11. As the helpers are mounting the strips, have the rest of the class follow these cleanup instructions (also on pg. 57 of the Student Activity Book).

    - Put the envelope of unused protein test papers in the storage bag.
    - Flush the developing solution of alcohol and vinegar down the drain.
    - Empty and rinse out the dropper bottles of cornstarch, corn syrup, and milk. Also empty and rinse out the dropper bottle of corn oil, since you will not need it for the remaining lessons.
    - Wash, rinse, and dry the forceps and return them to the lab bag.
    - Wipe the test trays with paper towels, wash and rinse them out, and wipe them again.
    - Place the dropper bottles, test trays, and box of toothpicks in the liquids bag.
    - Throw out the used toothpicks and paper towels and return all materials to the storage bag.
    - Return the storage bag to the storage area.

    Note: Because the developing solution contains alcohol and vinegar—both biodegradable substances—it will not harm the water system.

Final Activities

1. Have a member from each group come up to the "Class Liquids Test Table" and write his or her group's test result for each liquid.

2. Then, starting with water, ask the class to describe what happened to the protein test papers with each liquid. Discuss any differing results and have students repeat the test later.

3. Have students look at their test results. Ask them which liquids contain protein and which do not.

4. Now have students look again at the class table and focus on all the results for water when it was tested for starch, glucose, fat, and protein. Give the groups a few minutes to review and discuss all the results for water. Ask if they can draw any conclusions about water. Then have groups share conclusions with the rest of the class.

5. Finally, have students write in their notebooks a few sentences about why they think our bodies need water.

    Note: Remind students to research their two questions about protein and to be ready to share answers in the next lesson.

Extensions

1. Separate the protein in milk by mixing the milk with vinegar and pouring the mixture through cheesecloth or a coffee filter to separate the curds and whey. Then students can use protein test papers to test each part. Which part has protein?

2. Suggest that students research one of the following topics about milk.

    - What are the many things that happen to milk between the time the cow is milked and the time the carton arrives on the grocery shelf? Have students draw a diagram to show all the steps.

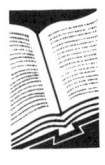

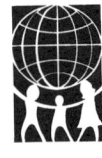

124 / Testing Liquids for Proteins

STC / *Food Chemistry*

LESSON 12

- What products come from milk? Ask students to make a poster to share with younger children.

- What jobs are involved in milk production? Have students find the name of the dairy from which the milk in a carton came and write a letter asking for information.

3. Have students touch the protein test papers with their fingers. Develop the test papers and talk about the results.

4. How are glucose test papers and protein test papers alike and different? Have students use a Venn diagram to draw comparisons.

5. Ask students to research water. Why is it important to our health? How much should we drink every day?

Assessments

In the three lessons of this cycle, look for growth in the following areas.

Lab Procedures

- Do students use forceps properly when handling the protein test papers?

- This is a more complicated test than previous ones. Are students following procedures correctly?

- Do students demonstrate competence with basic cleanup procedures?

Discussions

- Can students accurately describe their test results?

- Can students readily identify reasons for discrepant results?

- Do students conclude that water does not contain any of the nutrients identified in this unit?

- Do students discuss combinations of nutrients found in each food?

Written Work

- Are data tables improving in clarity and accuracy?

- Do notebook entries about water reflect ideas expressed during the class discussion?

- Do students indicate that test results may vary because there are different amounts of protein in each food?

Student Instructions for Testing Liquids for Proteins

1. Hold the test papers with the forceps to avoid contamination. Number the papers from one to five by writing a number on the white end. (Use a pencil to write the numbers.)

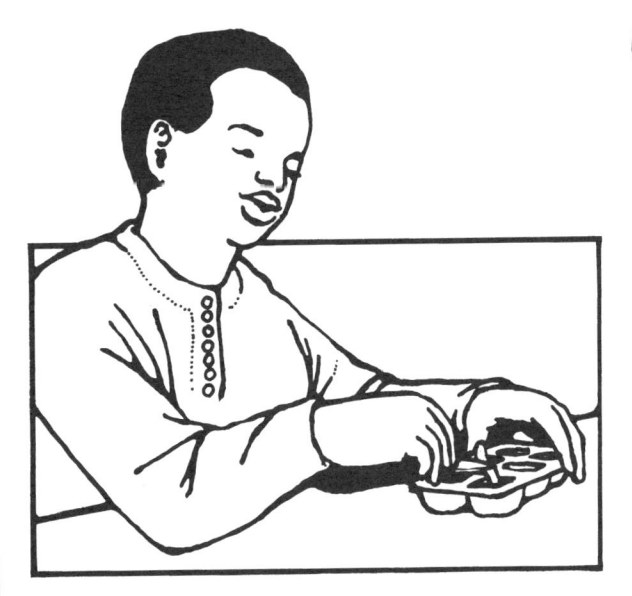

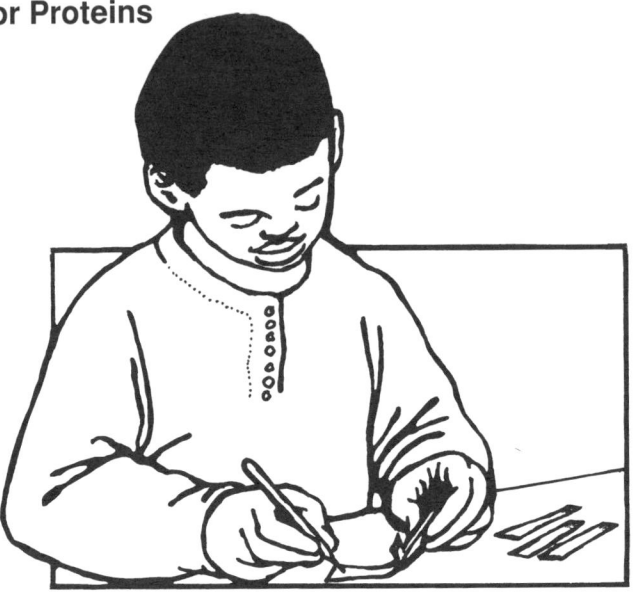

2. Put three drops of each liquid in its appropriate section of the test tray.

3. Then use the forceps to put an unnumbered protein test paper in the unnumbered section of your test tray. This is your control.

4. Using the forceps, put the blue end of each numbered protein test paper in each liquid just long enough to wet it.

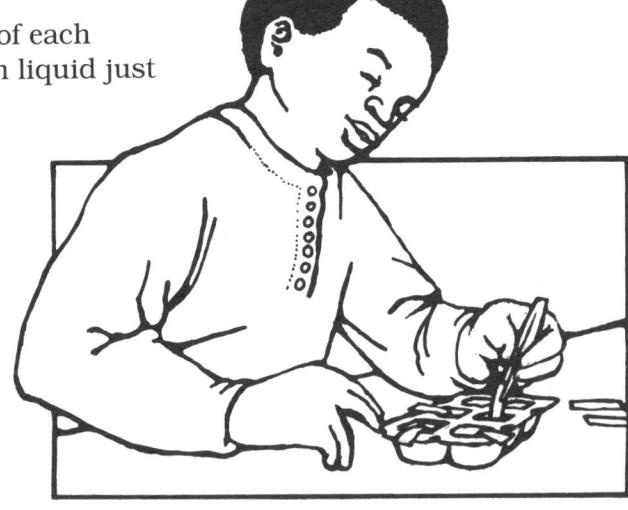

5. Remove each protein test paper from the test tray and blot off the extra liquid with a paper towel.

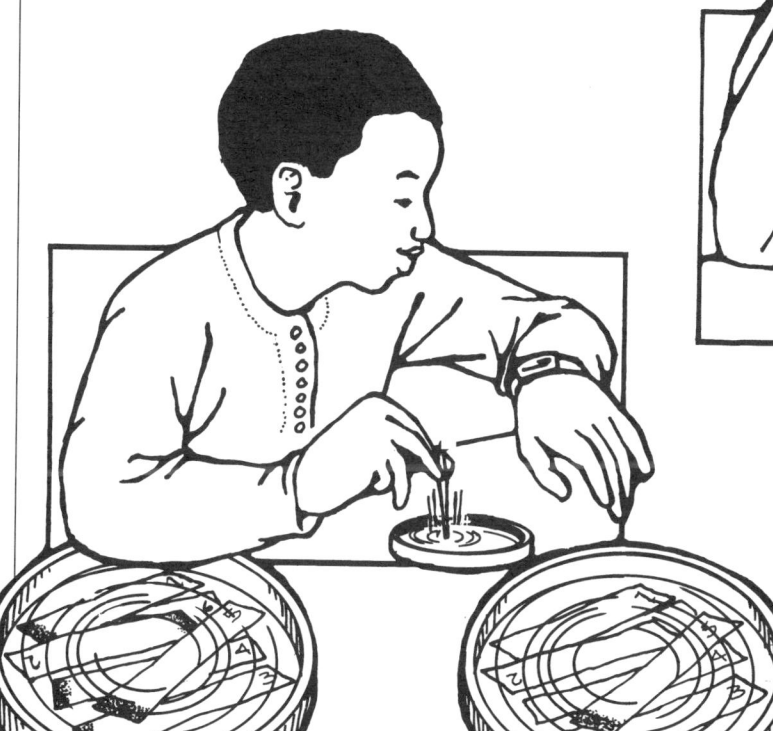

6. Soak all the protein test papers in the developing solution for about five minutes, stirring the solution gently with a toothpick. (It's okay to use one toothpick to do all the stirring.) Make sure the blue part of each test strip is completely covered with developing solution.

7. Wait five minutes for the papers to develop. Write in your notebook two questions about proteins you would like to answer.

8. After five minutes, remove all the protein test papers from the developing solution and put them on a paper towel to dry.

9. Tape the control to your liquids table for the proteins test. Then compare the other test papers to the control.

10. Follow the cleanup instructions.

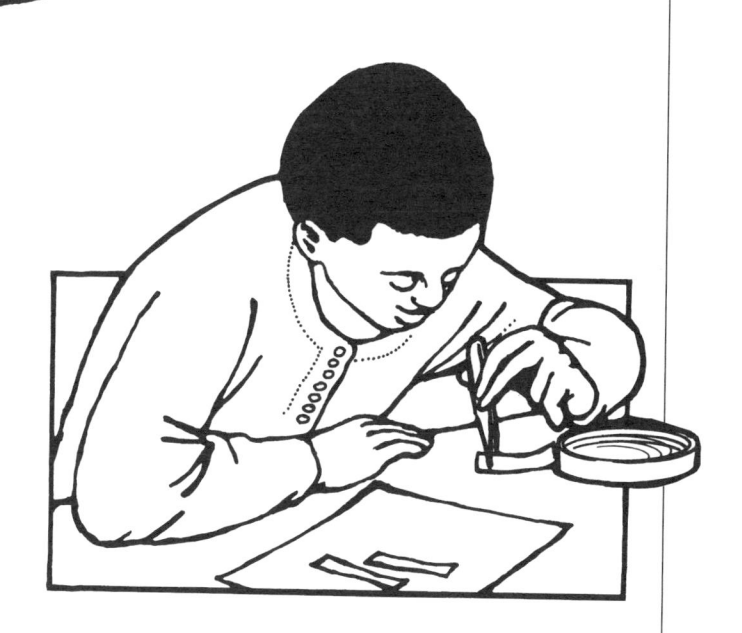

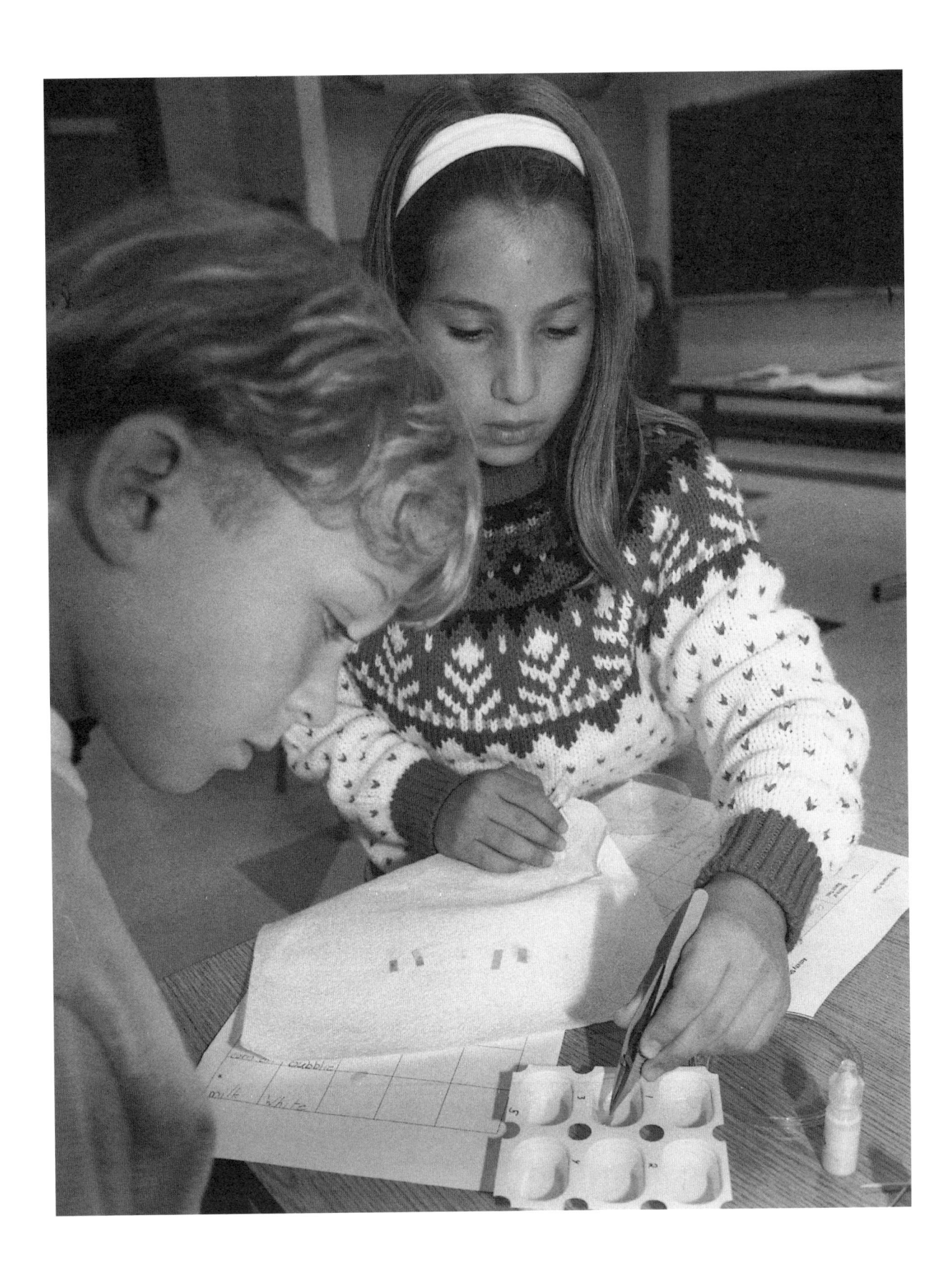

LESSON 13

Testing Foods for Proteins

Overview and Objectives

Now that students have learned a test for proteins, they will apply it to their foods. From this investigation, students will obtain a range of data indicating that the amount of protein in foods differs from food to food. As a consequence, students gain further experience in describing and interpreting a range of results.

- Students share with the class what they have learned about proteins through individual research.

- Students design a data table to record their results of testing foods for protein.

- Students make and record predictions of the foods they think do and do not contain proteins.

- Students apply the protein test to their foods, record and analyze results, and compare the range of results with their predictions.

- Students record and organize observations, discoveries, and questions about proteins and the test for proteins in their notebooks, and then they share these in a class discussion.

Background

Though results may vary to some degree, in general, you can expect the results in Figure 13-1 from this lesson's test.

Figure 13-1

Protein Test Results

Food	Protein Content	Protein Test Results
Peanuts and egg white	High	Blue color remains
Coconut	Medium	Blue color fades
Onion, rice, apple, flour, granola bar	Low	Blue color almost disappears

STC / *Food Chemistry*

LESSON 13

Materials

For each student
- 1 science notebook, including the individual liquids table for the protein test

For every four students
- 1 storage bag containing the following:
    - 1 envelope with 22 protein test papers
    - 1 food bag
    - 2 lab bags
    - 1 liquids bag
- 2 petri dishes
- 6 paper towels

For the class
- 1 plastic bottle of developing solution, 1 liter (1 qt)
- "Class Foods Test Table," from previous lessons, and large marker
- 8 notecards, 12.5 cm x 20 cm (5" x 8")
- 1 roll of clear plastic tape
- Cleanup materials (2 plastic-lined disposal boxes, sponges, paper towels)
- Soapy water (sink or buckets)
- Clear water (sink or buckets)

Figure 13-2

Many foods contain protein

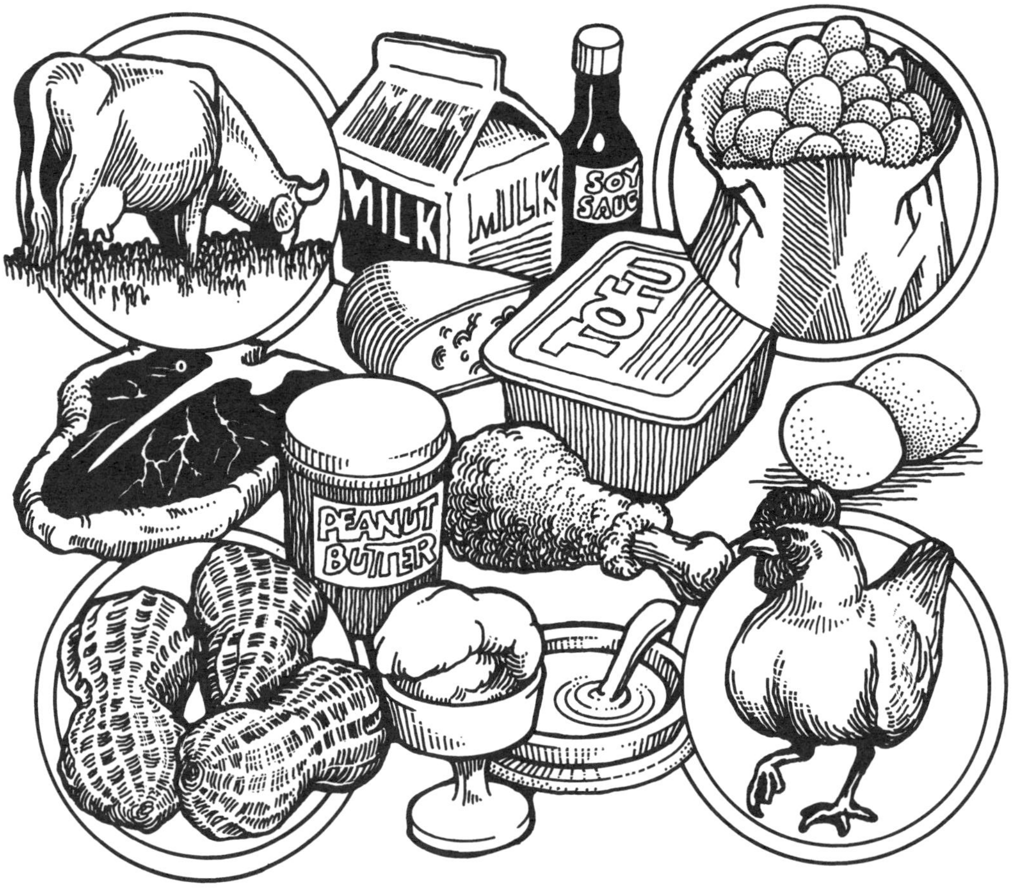

Preparation

1. If necessary, prepare more developing solution for the protein test papers. Mix together .5 liter (1 pt) of white vinegar and .5 liter (1 pt) of rubbing alcohol in the plastic quart mixing bottle. Store the solution in the closed bottle.

2. If necessary, have student helpers refill the dropper bottles of water used in Lesson 12.

Procedure

1. Ask students to share their questions and answers about proteins with their groups of four.

2. Then ask students to think about what they did in the last lesson and to suggest how they might test their foods for proteins.

3. Once again, have students construct their own foods test tables, this time for proteins. They may want to refer to earlier foods test tables for ideas on what to include.

4. Now ask students to predict for each food whether or not protein is present and to write the predictions on their tables. Ask some students to share the reasoning behind their predictions.

5. Briefly review the **Student Instructions for Testing Foods for Proteins** on pg. 133 in this guide and pg. 64 of the Student Activity Book.

   Note: Remind students to wipe the forceps carefully with a paper towel after each use with a different food.

6. Then have students pick up their test materials and sit with their groups. Ask a member from each group to pick up the following:
   - the group's storage bag
   - 2 petri dishes
   - 6 paper towels

7. Ask students to start testing. As they begin, pour into each flat dish just enough developing solution to cover the bottom completely.

   Note: Alert students that the developer solution may turn blue from the Coomassie blue on the test strips. (The developer is dissolving the Coomassie blue from the papers.) If this happens, discard the blue solution and add fresh solution.

8. After the papers are developed, ask students to record their observations on their tables. Make sure students are careful to describe the differences in intensity of blue for each food tested (for example, dark blue, light blue, very little blue; or, dark blue, faded blue, very faded blue, no blue). If colored pencils are available, students may also want to use coloring to illustrate the differences in color intensity. Remind them to save the protein test papers.

   Note: Point out that while there is a range of color intensity, test papers that retain any blue at all indicate the presence of some protein.

9. Ask students to lay the strips out on the paper towel in order from most blue to no blue. Have them review their tables to be sure this order matches the results they have recorded. Then have students look at the strips and list in their notebooks the foods in order from those containing the greatest amount of protein to those containing the least amount of protein.

LESSON 13

10. Now, one food at a time, collect the used protein test papers for each of the eight foods the whole class is testing. (Do not collect the used papers for the two foods students have brought from home). Ask student helpers to label a notecard and mount the results for each food, just as they did for the liquids. This will help the class interpret and compare results in Lesson 14.

11. As the students are mounting the strips, have the rest of the class follow these cleanup instructions (also on pg. 62 of the Student Activity Book).

    - Flush the developing solution down the drain.
    - Put the correct lids securely on the cups of food.
    - Return the dropper bottle of water to the liquids bag.
    - Discard the contents of the test trays and the used toothpicks into the plastic-lined disposal boxes.
    - Wipe the spoons with a paper towel and return the food cups and spoons to the food bag.
    - Wash the test trays in soapy water, rinse them in clean water, and wipe them dry.
    - Wash, rinse, and dry the forceps. Return them and the test trays to the lab bag.
    - Put the lab bags, food bag, and liquids bag back in the storage bag.
    - Return the materials to the storage area.

12. Finally, have a student from each group record the group's test results on the "Class Foods Test Table."

    Note: Save the mounted display of protein test papers for use in Lesson 14.

Final Activities

Ask students to write a few sentences in their notebooks answering the following questions:

- What did you do during this lesson?
- What did you discover?
- How did the results compare with your predictions?
- Using the list in your notebook, what conclusions can you draw about the amount of protein in the foods?

Management Tip: In Lesson 14, students will retest foods for protein if there were discrepant results. You will need to prepare envelopes of test strips and make sure you have enough developing solution for any retesting needed.

Extensions

1. Write a shape poem about a food that contains proteins.
2. Plan a class indoor or outdoor picnic that includes five different sources of proteins.
3. Ask students to use their tables, record sheets, notebook entries, research, and reading selections to make up questions about food chemistry. Have students record each question on an index card. Collect the cards and use them to play a quiz game.

Student Instructions for Testing Foods for Proteins

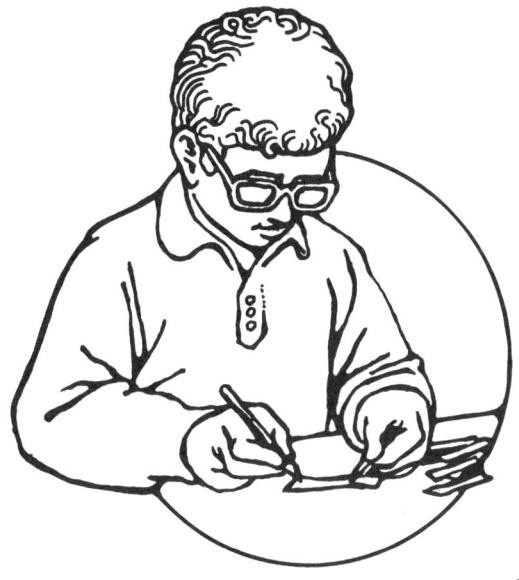

1. Hold the protein test papers with forceps to avoid contamination. Number ten test papers from one to ten by writing the number on the white end. (Use a pencil to write the numbers.)

2. Put a spoonful of rice in section 1 of your ten-section test tray. Let the rice soak in several drops of water while you prepare the remaining foods.

3. As with the starch and glucose tests, some foods need preparation before testing. You and your partner may use your fingers to shell the peanut since you will not be touching the actual food. (Touching the test food with your fingers may contaminate the foods.) Use your forceps to place a shelled peanut or two and small portions of dried apple and granola into their matching numbered sections of the test tray. Then, also with forceps, do the following:
   - Tear the apple into small pieces.
   - Remove the peanut's papery skin. Hold down the peanut with forceps and have your partner use the other forceps to crumble the kernel.
   - Crumble a small piece of the granola bar.

4. Put a small spoonful of each of the other foods into your test tray. Make sure the number of each spoon matches the number of the food and the test tray section you put it in.

5. Put two or three drops of water on each food in the tray. Using different toothpicks, stir each food for about a minute until it is wet.

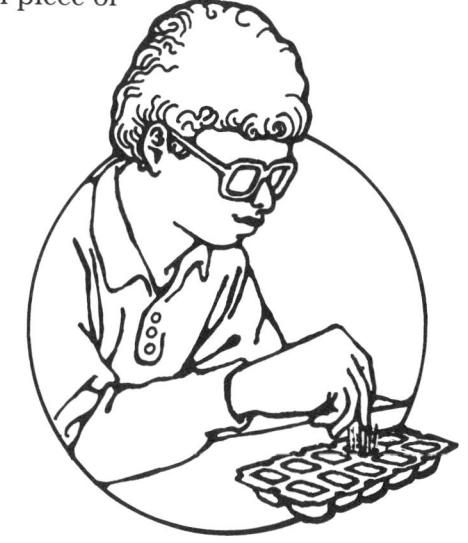

6. Using forceps, place the unnumbered protein test paper on a paper towel. This is your control.

LESSON 13

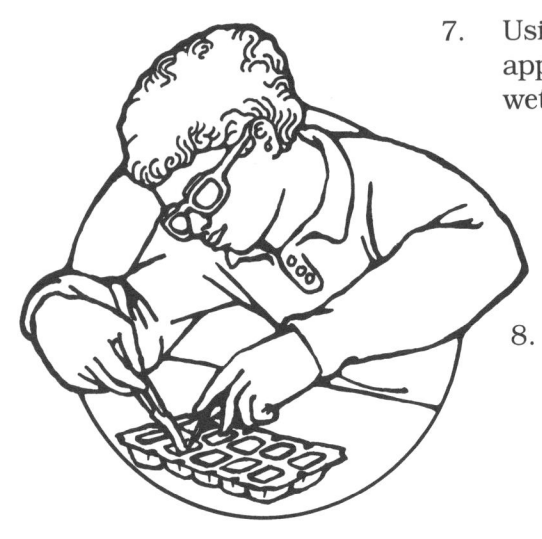

7. Using forceps, dip the blue end of the appropriately numbered test paper in the wet part of the egg white.

   For the other foods, use a toothpick to mash a bit of the dampened food onto the blue part of the appropriately numbered test paper.

8. With toothpicks, brush off any extra food from each test paper. With a paper towel, blot off any extra liquid.

9. Using forceps, place all the protein test papers in the developing solution so that the blue tip is in the solution.

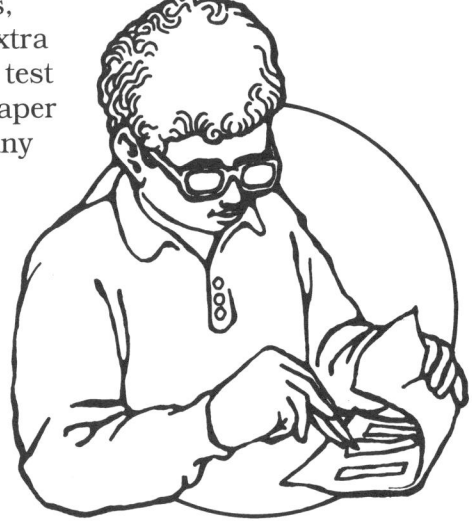

10. Leave the test papers in the developing solution for five minutes. Use a toothpick to keep stirring the papers around in the liquid.

11. After five minutes, remove the protein test papers from the developing solution and place them on a paper towel in order from most blue to no blue. After they dry, your teacher will collect them.

12. Compare results with your control. Also look at your results from the liquids test for proteins.

13. Discuss observations with your teammates and record them on your foods table.

14. Now follow your cleanup instructions.

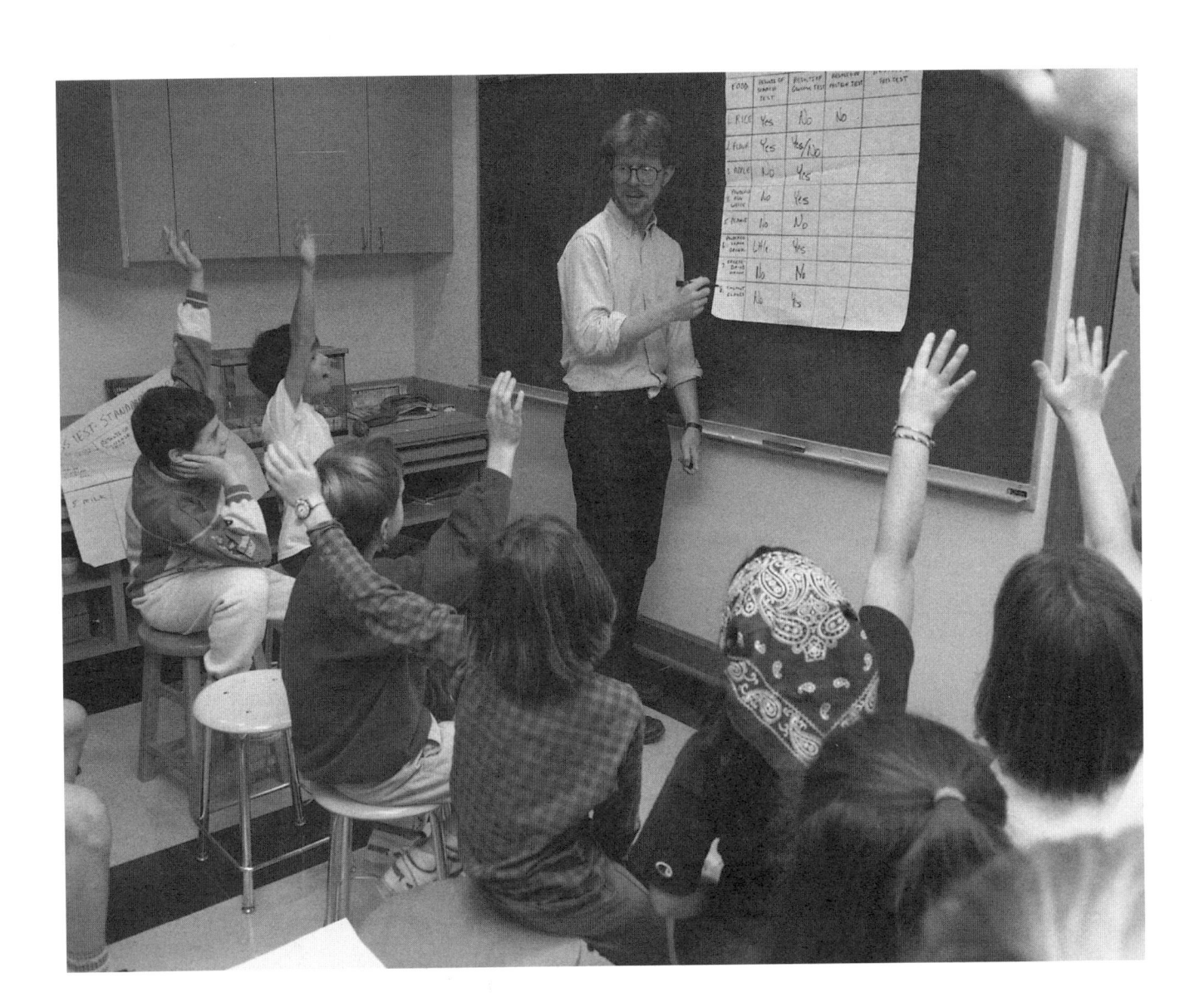

LESSON 14

Learning More about Proteins

Overview and Objectives

In this lesson, students' analysis of their data and a class discussion reinforce the understanding that many different kinds of food contain proteins, and in varying amounts. Students also discover that many foods, including some they have tested, contain more than one nutrient and that they can use this new knowledge to help them decide which foods to eat in order to maintain sound nutrition.

- Students analyze and discuss the protein test results of the class as a whole and retest foods for which test results differed.

- Students create Venn diagrams of the different nutrients in their test foods and discuss the relationship between nutrients and healthy foods.

- Students read about proteins as an important part of diet.

- Students apply what they have learned about starch, glucose, fats, and proteins to solve a hypothetical problem.

Background

The **Reading Selection** on pg. 140 presents more information about proteins and their essential role in our diet. Once again, it is useful to remind students that our scientific knowledge about diet will continue to grow. As it does, new information will appear in daily newspapers and in magazine articles. Students can also stay tuned in to nutrition-related issues by watching or listening to the news.

Materials

For each student
- 1 science notebook, including the individual foods table for the protein test from Lesson 13

For every four students
- 1 sheet of newsprint
- 1 large marker

For retesting, if needed
- 1 storage bag containing the following:
    - 1 food bag
    - 2 lab bags
    - 1 liquids bag

STC / *Food Chemistry*

LESSON 14

    2 petri dishes
    4 paper towels
       Extra protein test papers

For the class
    "Class Foods Test Table," from previous lessons
    "Questions We Have about Foods" list and large marker
    Mounted protein test papers from Lesson 13

Preparation

1. Post the "Class Foods Test Table." Make sure the "Questions We Have about Foods" list is also posted.
2. Put the mounted protein test papers from Lesson 13 in a visible place.
3. Read "Proteins: The Building Blocks of Life," on pg. 140.

Procedure

1. Ask students to share what they learned about the proteins in their foods. Encourage them to use their individual food test tables, notebook entries, the "Class Foods Test Table," and the mounted display of the protein test papers.
2. If students have obtained different results, ask them to explain briefly why this may have happened and how the class can determine whether or not the food in question actually does contain some protein.
3. Give students time to retest foods for which results differed (refer to pgs. 130 to 131 in Lesson 13 for materials and preparation needed).
4. Then ask students to work in their groups to create Venn diagrams that organize the foods on the basis of the nutrients they contain. Each student should draw these Venn diagrams in his or her notebook. (Figure 14-1 shows one example of the type of Venn diagrams students may draw.)
5. Have them use the Venn diagrams to answer in their notebooks the following questions:
   - Which foods contained all four nutrients?
   - Which foods contained none of the nutrients for which you tested?
   - Which of the foods you tested do you now think are "healthy"? Why?
6. Have students look back to the entries they made in their notebooks in Lesson 2. Has their thinking changed? Encourage them to discuss why or why not.

Final Activities

1. Ask students to read "Proteins: The Building Blocks of Life," on pg. 69 in the Student Activity Book.
2. Then ask students to work in their groups of four to solve the following problem. Have them gather data from their tables, notebook entries, and reading selections for help.
   - If you were going on an all-day hike, which food (or foods) on the class table would you take with you and why? Include at least three good reasons.

LESSON 14

Figure 14-1

Sample Venn diagram

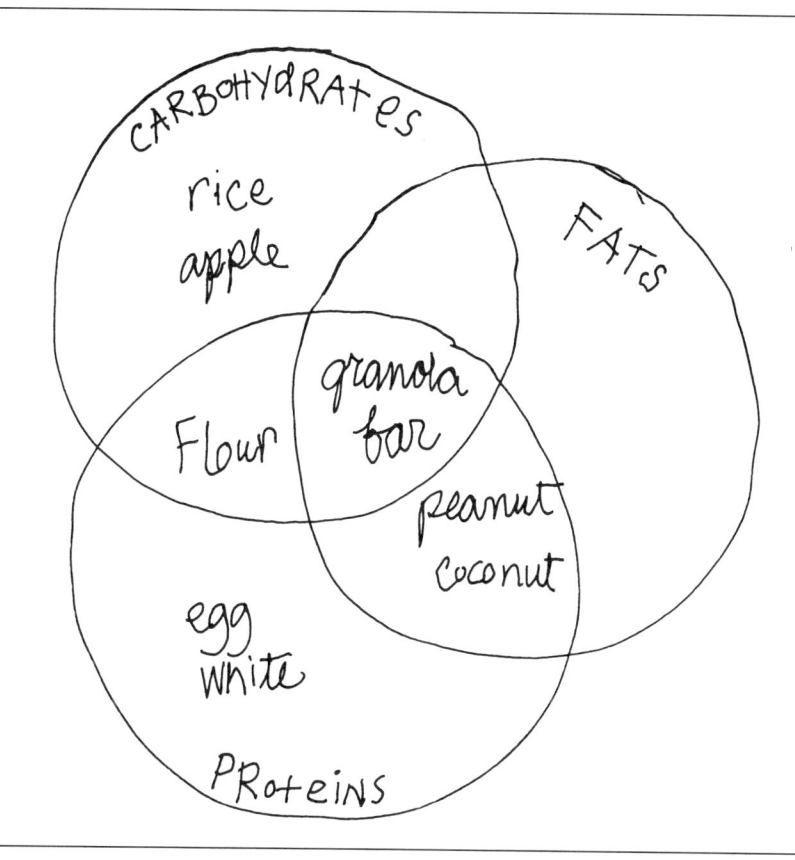

[Venn diagram with four overlapping circles labeled CARBOHYDRATES (containing rice, apple), FATS, PROTEINS (containing egg white), with Flour in carbohydrates/proteins overlap, granola bar in center, peanut and coconut in fats/proteins overlap]

3. Give each group a marker and piece of newsprint on which to write their ideas. Have each group choose a spokesperson to report back to the class.

4. Remind students to add any new questions to the "Questions We Have about Foods" list.

Extensions

1. Hold a vegetarian recipe "swap" or a vegetarian lunch day.

2. Remind the class that proteins come from both plants and animals. Have the class brainstorm a list of plant sources and a list of animal sources.

Assessments

To help you assess student growth, you may want to refer back to the **Assessments** section on pg. 125 of Lesson 12.

LESSON 14

Reading Selection

Proteins: The Building Blocks of Life

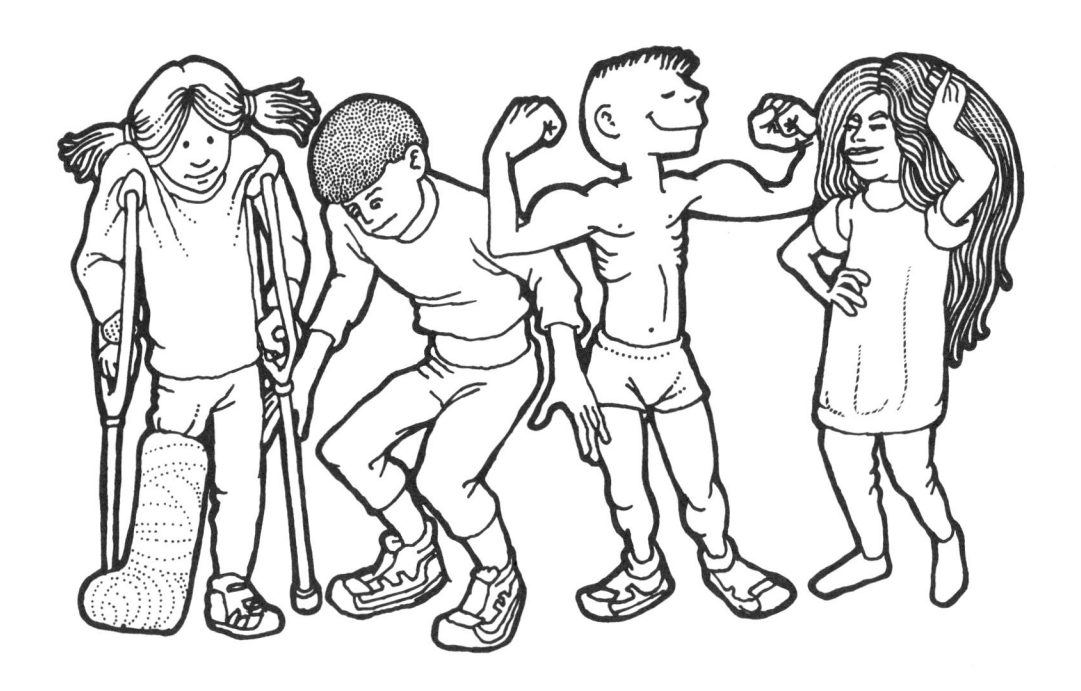

Proteins are your body's building blocks, the stuff that helps your body grow and repair itself. Most of the material in your skin, hair, muscles, and organs (such as your heart and kidneys) is made up of proteins. For months before you were even born, proteins were used for building your body. They will continue to build and repair your tissues for the rest of your life.

In this day and age, Americans get their protein from a variety of sources, including eggs, milk, cheese, meat, fish, cereal grains, and legumes. There has always been plenty of protein in this country, but actually getting it to the dinner table hasn't always been easy.

Buffalo for Dinner

In the old days, Native Americans and pioneers couldn't go to the supermarket to buy beef, eggs, or milk. They had to hunt for protein or trade with somebody else. Instead of eating a lot of beef, Native Americans ate wild animals like deer, turkey, rabbit, and buffalo.

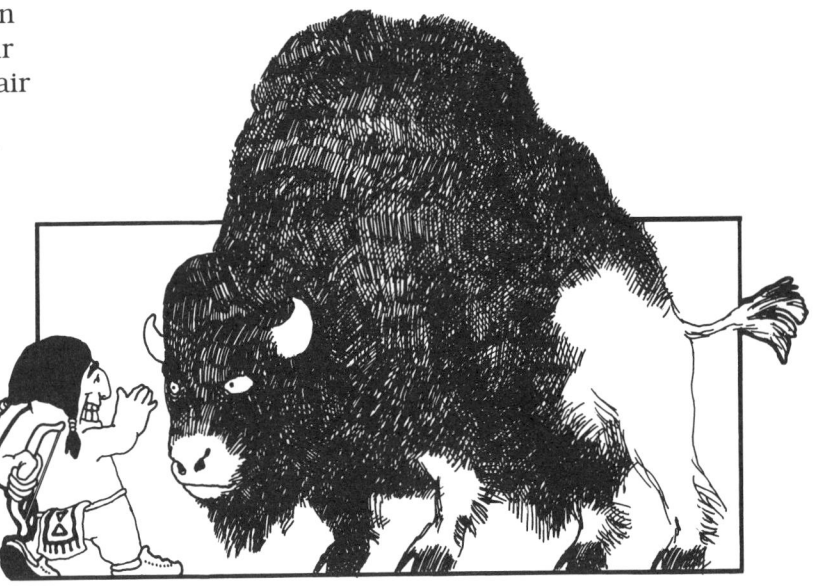

Pioneers ate these things too. But when they settled down and built their own homesteads, they began to raise chickens and pigs. Pioneers also milked cows every day and got some protein from milk and the cheese they made from it. But before refrigerators, it was hard to keep milk products fresh for more than a day or two.

In the second half of the 19th century, beef cattle became a major industry in the West. (Where do you think the term "cowboy" came from?) America became one of the biggest meat-eating nations in the world. By the late 1960s, 30% of the American diet was meat, while in most other countries, people were eating less meat than that, getting more of their protein from fish or certain vegetables.

Even today, most Americans eat more protein than they need. And much of that comes from meat. For example, think about a single hamburger. That's about three or four ounces of meat, and it's enough protein to satisfy daily growth needs for most of us. But we can see that many Americans eat far more meat than that.

This could be a problem, because some research findings show that eating too much red meat (and the fat it often contains) may not be healthy. So, instead, more people are trying to eat more fish and poultry, which contain protein but often less fat. Some Americans are vegetarians, and, like many other people around the world, have stopped eating all meats. To stay healthy, vegetarians must plan their diets carefully and eat a wide variety of foods that contain protein.

Anyone for Tofu?
That's really not so hard, either. For one thing, legumes—including beans, peas, and peanuts—are a great source of protein. Because they're so inexpensive, beans have been called "the poor man's meat." But there's nothing poor about the amount of proteins legumes pack. A bowl of thick minestrone soup or a peanut butter sandwich can provide as much protein as a hamburger, omelet, or piece of chicken.

The soybean is especially useful. Soybeans produce more protein per acre than any other plant or animal. They're easy to grow and can be made to taste like other foods. You may already have eaten soy mixed in hamburger or cereal and not even known it!

And a soy product called tofu is becoming more popular (you can probably find it in your local supermarket). Tofu is the "chameleon" of foods. It can be used in salads, casseroles, quiches, burgers, and stews, and it can even be made into a food that tastes like ice cream.

As you can see, the amounts and types of protein we eat have changed over time. But the human need for protein hasn't changed a bit. And while we don't need a lot of protein to stay healthy, we do need some. So for now, our best bet may be to eat a variety of protein foods from both plants and animals.

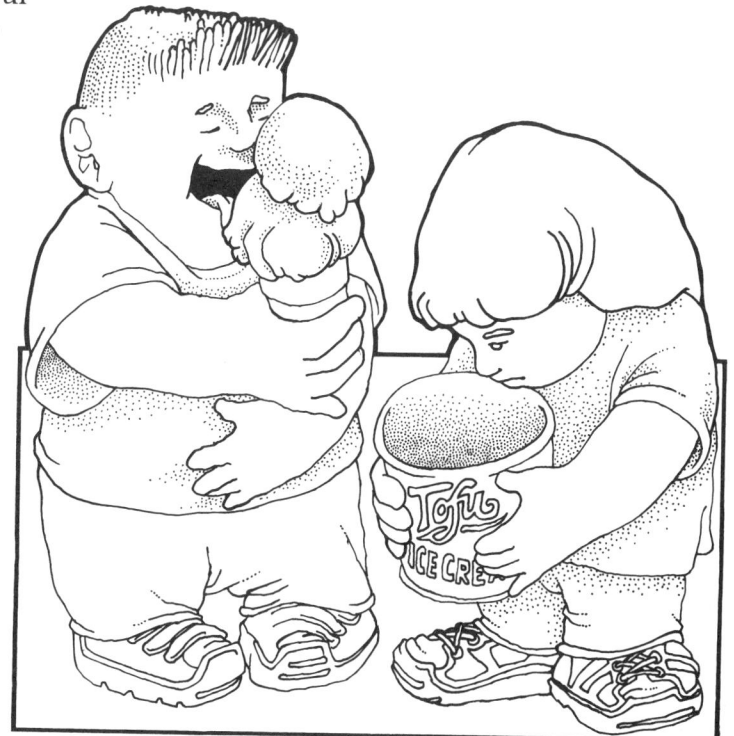

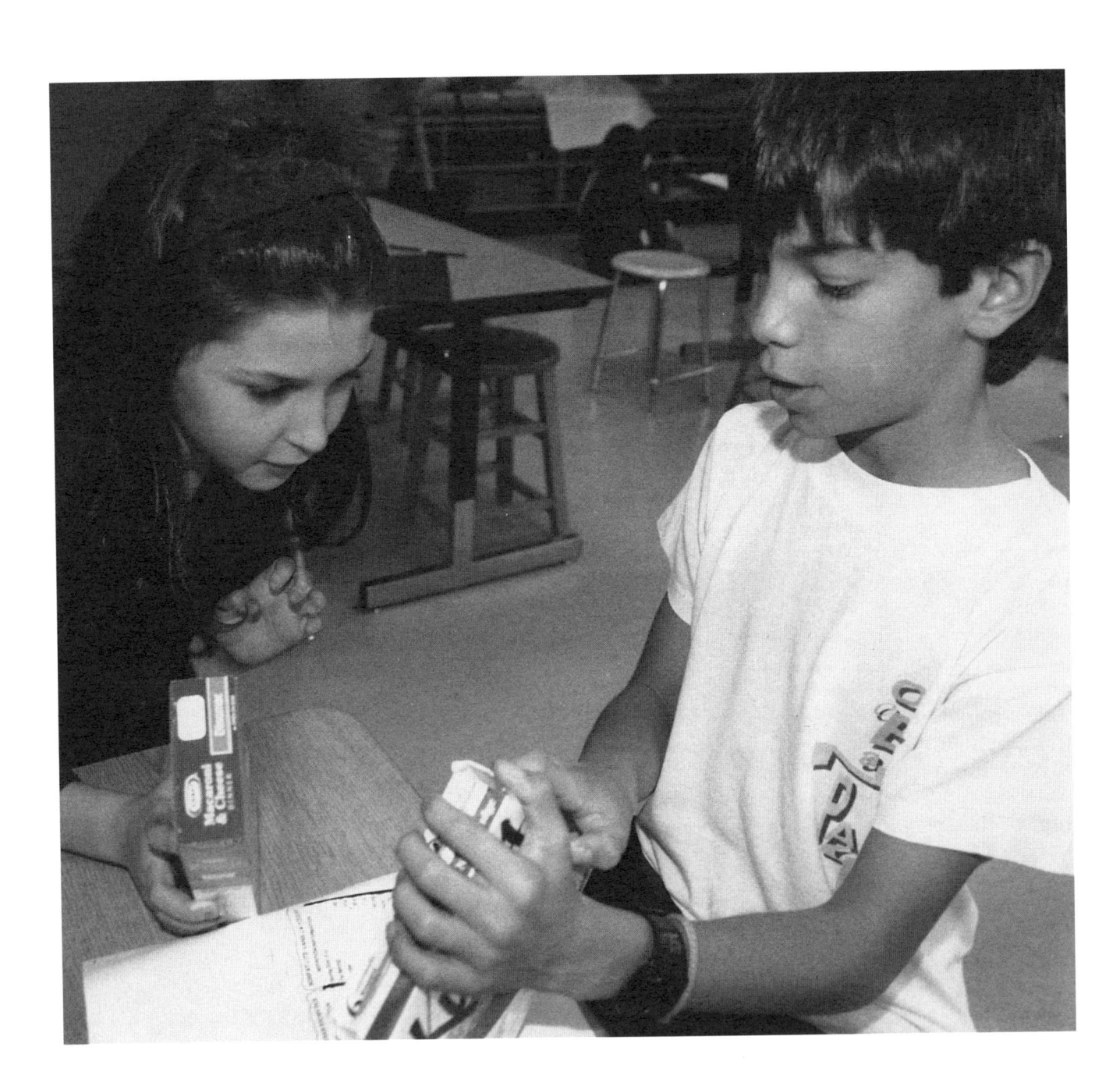

LESSON 15

Examining Labels: Making the Connection

Overview and Objectives

In this lesson, students find out more about the nutrients in the foods they eat by reading food labels. They are given the opportunity to connect their test data to the information on food labels, but they also discover that food labels can give them information they cannot get from their tests. Students will find some vitamins listed on the labels, and they are given the chance to think about the importance of this type of nutrient, too.

- Students identify and interpret the information on a food label.

- Students compare the nutrient information from their foods test results with the nutrient information on labels for those foods.

- Students read about several vitamins and discuss why information about certain vitamins is listed on food labels.

Background

In 1990, Congress passed the Nutrition Labeling and Education Act, which requires the Food and Drug Administration (FDA) to develop new standards for labels on all packaged foods. The new label is designed to give consumers information for making healthy choices regarding their total daily diet. An example of the label appears in Figure 15-1.

Other changes in the new label standards include the following:

- A food can be described as "light" or "lite" only if it has 50% less fat or sodium than the food to which it is compared.

- The word "more" can be used only if the food contains 10% more of a given ingredient than the foods to which it is being compared (for example, "more raisins than any other cereal").

- Solid scientific research must support any health claim linking specific diseases to dietary excesses or deficits.

The calories listed on the label are the calories people often talk about when they are watching their weight. A calorie is the amount of energy required to raise the temperature of 1 cubic centimeter of water by 1° Celsius. The number of calories in a serving of food represents the amount of energy our bodies can get from that food and also how much energy the body will store if we don't use that energy right away.

LESSON 15

Figure 15-1

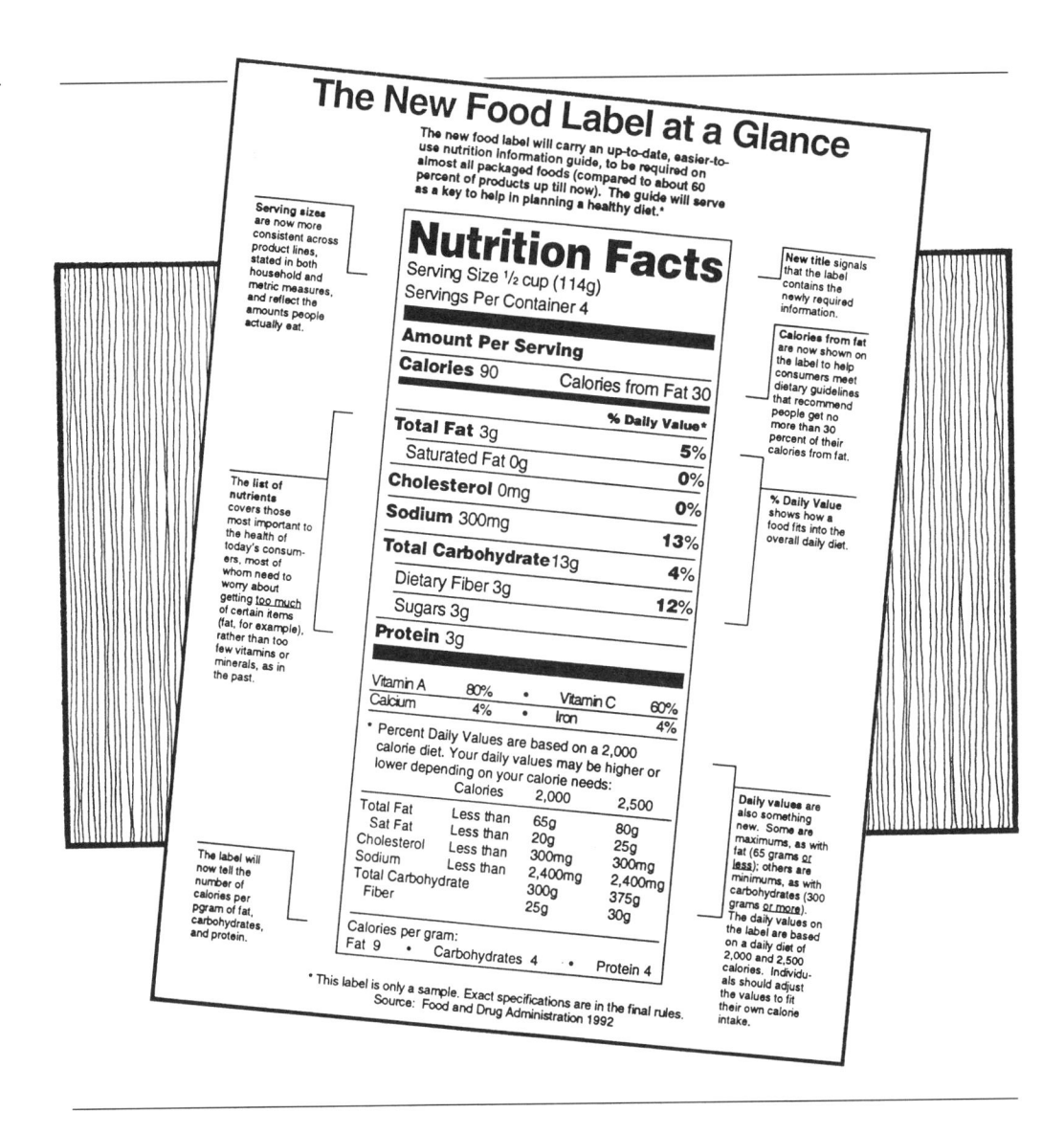

The New Food Label at a Glance

The new food label will carry an up-to-date, easier-to-use nutrition information guide, to be required on almost all packaged foods (compared to about 60 percent of products up till now). The guide will serve as a key to help in planning a healthy diet.*

Nutrition Facts
Serving Size ½ cup (114g)
Servings Per Container 4

Amount Per Serving	
Calories 90	Calories from Fat 30

	% Daily Value*
Total Fat 3g	5%
Saturated Fat 0g	0%
Cholesterol 0mg	0%
Sodium 300mg	13%
Total Carbohydrate 13g	4%
Dietary Fiber 3g	12%
Sugars 3g	
Protein 3g	

Vitamin A	80%	•	Vitamin C	60%
Calcium	4%	•	Iron	4%

* Percent Daily Values are based on a 2,000 calorie diet. Your daily values may be higher or lower depending on your calorie needs:

	Calories	2,000	2,500
Total Fat	Less than	65g	80g
Sat Fat	Less than	20g	25g
Cholesterol	Less than	300mg	300mg
Sodium	Less than	2,400mg	2,400mg
Total Carbohydrate		300g	375g
Fiber		25g	30g

Calories per gram:
Fat 9 • Carbohydrates 4 • Protein 4

* This label is only a sample. Exact specifications are in the final rules.
Source: Food and Drug Administration 1992

Serving sizes are now more consistent across product lines, stated in both household and metric measures, and reflect the amounts people actually eat.

The list of nutrients covers those most important to the health of today's consumers, most of whom need to worry about getting too much of certain items (fat, for example), rather than too few vitamins or minerals, as in the past.

The label will now tell the number of calories per gram of fat, carbohydrates, and protein.

New title signals that the label contains the newly required information.

Calories from fat are now shown on the label to help consumers meet dietary guidelines that recommend people get no more than 30 percent of their calories from fat.

% Daily Value shows how a food fits into the overall daily diet.

Daily values are also something new. Some are maximums, as with fat (65 grams or less); others are minimums, as with carbohydrates (300 grams or more). The daily values on the label are based on a daily diet of 2,000 and 2,500 calories. Individuals should adjust the values to fit their own calorie intake.

The connection between calories and weight lies in the body's storage of calories, or energy not yet used. Our body stores that energy in the form of glycogen first and then fat. The more we eat that we don't need, the more fat gets stored and potentially added as unwanted weight.

Now that students know about different nutrients and their importance in the diet, they can use labels to find out which nutrients are in the packaged foods they eat. In addition, students can use labels to compare different commercial foods for the nutritional content and value and to help them make informed choices about their dietary habits.

Note: The labels students use in this lesson (see pgs. 158 and 159) come from food packages available at the time *Food Chemistry* was written. New regulations from the FDA or other federal agencies may cause food labels to change over time.

LESSON 15

Materials

For each student
- 1 science notebook
- 1 **Record Sheet 15-A, Comparing Test Results and Food Labels**
- 1 corn flakes label (either from pg. 72 in the Student Activity Book or copied from the blackline master on pg. 158 of this guide)

For every four students
- 4 labels (copied from the blackline master on pg. 159)
- 1 No. 1 paper clip

For the class
- "Class Foods Test Table"
- Newsprint or poster board and large marker, or overhead transparency and pen

Preparation

1. Make one copy of **Record Sheet 15-A, Comparing Test Results and Food Labels** for each student.

2. If students do not have the Student Activity Book, copy one corn flakes label (see pg. 158) for each student.

3. Prepare one copy of the sheet of four labels on pg. 159 for each group of four students.

4. Have student helpers cut each label page into four labels and paper clip them together.

Procedure

1. Begin by asking students if they can think of another way, besides testing, to determine the nutrient content of foods. If they do not suggest reading food labels, raise the idea. Ask students to share what they know about the information on food labels. Record their ideas on newsprint or an overhead transparency. Or, ask students to record ideas quickly in their notebooks.

2. Now pass out copies of the corn flakes label (see Figure 15-2) or have students look at the label on pg. 72 of the Student Activity Book. Ask the class what information is given and list responses on a sheet of newsprint.

3. Next, explain that students will compare the information from their test results for four of the eight foods tested by the whole class (rice, granola bar, peanuts, and flour) with the information on the food labels for these foods. Pass out **Record Sheet 15-A, Comparing Test Results and Food Labels** and a bundle of four food labels to each group of four.

4. Explain that each student will be responsible for one of the food labels. Ask the groups to decide which of the four foods each member will be responsible for and to write that food on the top of his or her Record Sheet. Then ask students to use their own test tables and the "Class Foods Test Table" to complete **Record Sheet 15-A**.

   Note: As students begin to analyze food labels, they are likely to raise many questions such as "What is a gram?" "What is sodium?" and "What is fiber?" Extension 2 at the end of this lesson offers suggestions on how students can answer these questions.

LESSON 15

Figure 15-2

A sample corn flakes label

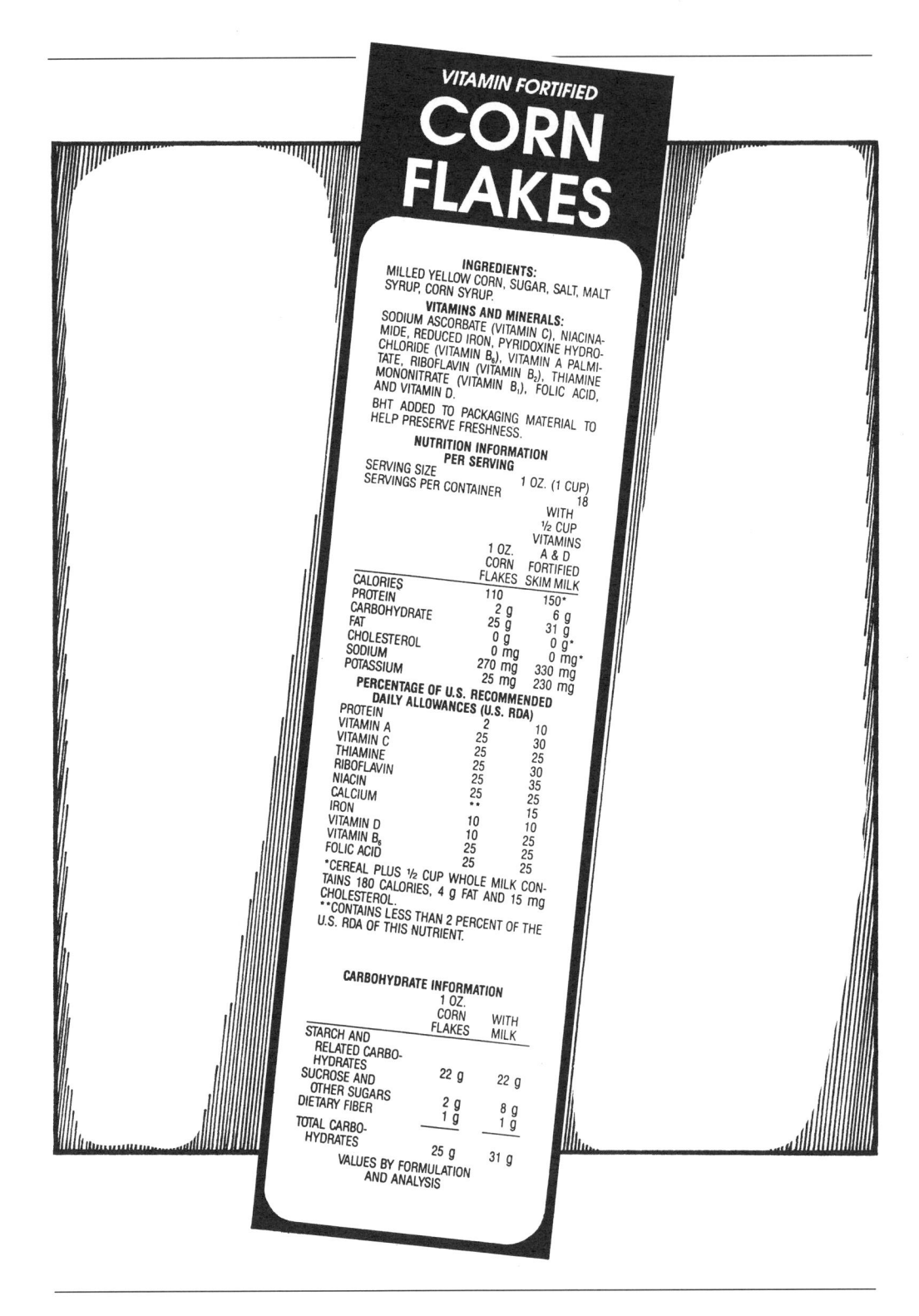

VITAMIN FORTIFIED CORN FLAKES

INGREDIENTS:
MILLED YELLOW CORN, SUGAR, SALT, MALT SYRUP, CORN SYRUP.

VITAMINS AND MINERALS:
SODIUM ASCORBATE (VITAMIN C), NIACINAMIDE, REDUCED IRON, PYRIDOXINE HYDROCHLORIDE (VITAMIN B_6), VITAMIN A PALMITATE, RIBOFLAVIN (VITAMIN B_2), THIAMINE MONONITRATE (VITAMIN B_1), FOLIC ACID, AND VITAMIN D.

BHT ADDED TO PACKAGING MATERIAL TO HELP PRESERVE FRESHNESS.

NUTRITION INFORMATION PER SERVING

SERVING SIZE 1 OZ. (1 CUP)
SERVINGS PER CONTAINER 18

	1 OZ. CORN FLAKES	WITH ½ CUP VITAMINS A & D FORTIFIED SKIM MILK
CALORIES	110	150*
PROTEIN	2 g	6 g
CARBOHYDRATE	25 g	31 g
FAT	0 g	0 g*
CHOLESTEROL	0 mg	0 mg*
SODIUM	270 mg	330 mg
POTASSIUM	25 mg	230 mg

PERCENTAGE OF U.S. RECOMMENDED DAILY ALLOWANCES (U.S. RDA)

PROTEIN	2	10
VITAMIN A	25	30
VITAMIN C	25	25
THIAMINE	25	30
RIBOFLAVIN	25	35
NIACIN	25	25
CALCIUM	**	15
IRON	10	10
VITAMIN D	10	25
VITAMIN B_6	25	25
FOLIC ACID	25	25

*CEREAL PLUS ½ CUP WHOLE MILK CONTAINS 180 CALORIES, 4 g FAT AND 15 mg CHOLESTEROL.

**CONTAINS LESS THAN 2 PERCENT OF THE U.S. RDA OF THIS NUTRIENT.

CARBOHYDRATE INFORMATION

	1 OZ. CORN FLAKES	WITH MILK
STARCH AND RELATED CARBOHYDRATES	22 g	22 g
SUCROSE AND OTHER SUGARS	2 g	8 g
DIETARY FIBER	1 g	1 g
TOTAL CARBOHYDRATES	25 g	31 g

VALUES BY FORMULATION AND ANALYSIS

---

5. When students have completed their Record Sheets, have the class discuss how the information on the labels compares with the data from students' test results. For each food, ask students to discuss the following questions:

   ■ What information is alike?

   ■ What information is different?

LESSON 15

- What information did you learn from the label that you did not know from your test?

6. Ask students to write a few sentences in their notebooks explaining how food labels can help them make choices about what foods to eat.

Management Tip: You may wish to incorporate the **Final Activities** into your language arts period.

Final Activities

1. Ask students to look at their labels and find out what information is given about vitamins. Explain that vitamins are another important nutrient.

2. Then, using the following directions, have students read about vitamins. The **Reading Selections** begin on pg. 150 of this guide and on pg. 74 of the Student Activity Book.

    - Arrange students in groups of four.
    - Assign one vitamin to each group member.
    - Have all students assigned to the same vitamin meet to read and discuss the information.
    - Ask students to return to their groups of four and take turns teaching each other about the vitamin they have studied.

3. After students have shared information about each vitamin, hold a class discussion about why food labels contain information about vitamins.

Extensions

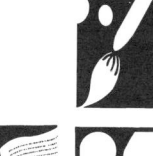

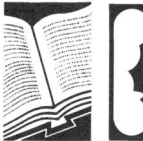

1. Give students a blank **Record Sheet 15-A, Comparing Test Results and Food Labels** to take home. Ask them to find labels for the test foods they brought from home and to record the label information. Then have students complete the table with their test results and compare the two sets of data.

2. Ask students to look at food labels at home and identify words that are not familiar. Have students research what the words mean and how they relate to foods and nutrition. Then have them report their findings to the class.

3. Have students compare the labels on a variety of cereal boxes and decide which cereal they think is the most nutritious. Ask the class to debate the nutritional pros and cons of several cereals.

4. Have students examine several different cereal boxes to determine the price, weight, and serving size for each cereal. Challenge them to use this information to solve practical problems. For example, have them compute the cost of cereal per ounce or gram. Then have each student decide what his or her own serving size actually is and compute its actual cost and nutritional value.

5. Challenge students to create an appealing new snack food by combining several foods from home. Have them design an appropriate box and logo and complete the nutritional information panel.

6. Have students research vitamins not described in the **Reading Selections** and share their findings with the class.

LESSON 15

Assessments

Discussions
- Can students identify ways their test data and food labels are alike?
- Can students identify information that is not available through their testing but is given on food labels?
- Can students clearly communicate information about a vitamin to other members of their group?
- Can students identify reasons why they think information about certain vitamins is listed on labels and information about other vitamins is not?

Written Work
- Do students refer to earlier test results (either individual or class) to complete **Record Sheet 15-A, Comparing Test Results and Food Labels**?
- Can students interpret and transfer information from the food labels to their table?
- Can students clearly communicate how food labels can help them make choices about the foods they eat?

Management Tip: Lesson 16 involves the testing of one food, marshmallows, for each of the four main nutrients studied in this unit. Appropriate testing materials for starch, glucose, fats, and protein must be prepared. You may want to review directions in previous lessons.

Record Sheet 15-A

Name: _____

Date: _____

LESSON 15

Comparing Test Results and Food Labels

Food: _____

Comparing Test Results and Food Labels Table

Nutrient	Test Results	Label
Carbohydrates		
Fats		
Proteins		

List the food's ingredients: _____

_____

STC / *Food Chemistry*

Reading Selections: Vitamins

Vitamin C: Scurvy No More

Think back to the days of tall sailing ships. Did you know one of the greatest dangers a sailor faced was getting sick from a disease called scurvy? It's true. Of course, warships and pirates were dangerous too. Even so, scurvy was one of a sailor's worst enemies. It could make a sailor's gums bleed, give him large black sores on his body, and make him extremely weak. Many men died from scurvy.

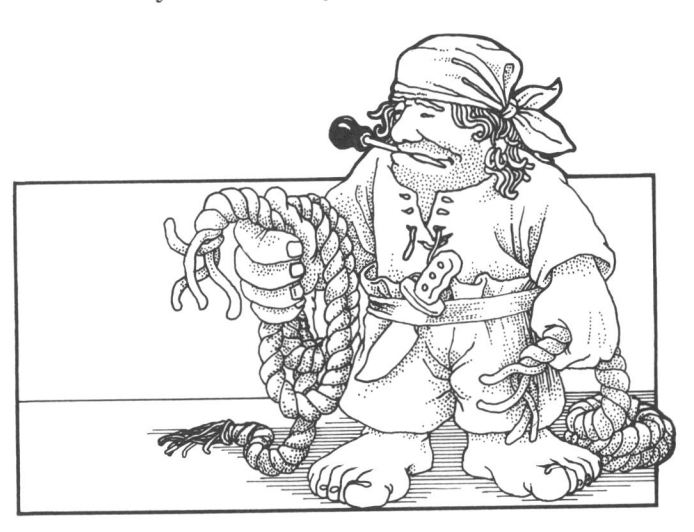

In the mid 1700s, a Scottish doctor named James Lind became interested in scurvy when he sailed with a British warship called the *Salisbury*. After three months of patrolling the southern coast of England, several crew members died of scurvy. All were sailors. None were officers.

Lind suspected that the cause of scurvy was related to food or to the crowded, dark, damp conditions on the ship. Lind observed that the officers ate meat, dried vegetables, and fruits. The crew ate salted meat, dried biscuits, butter, and small amounts of dried beans. He also observed that sailors slept under extremely crowded conditions in the lower decks of the ship.

Lind decided to collect more information about scurvy. He learned that French explorers in North America had once recovered from scurvy by drinking a broth of pine needles given to them by Iroquois Indians. He also heard about some Dutch sailors traveling on a boat full of citrus fruit. The Dutchmen came down with scurvy but quickly recovered after eating some of their cargo. Lind decided to conduct some diet-related tests.

A Surprising Cure

The doctor selected twelve sailors sick with scurvy and supplemented their diets. Every day, two were given apple cider; two were given spoonfuls of vinegar; two were given garlic and mustard herbs; two were given salt water; two were given sulfuric acid and alcohol with ginger and cinnamon; and two were given oranges and lemons.

The two sailors who ate the citrus fruit recovered quickly. They were even healthy enough to return to work within a few days. Lind decided he was onto something. He suggested that the British Navy begin giving its sailors a daily dose of lemon juice.

But the British Navy was not convinced that Lind's experiment proved anything. After all, how could fruit juice prevent a serious disease like scurvy? Naval officials just chalked up the sailors' recovery to coincidence and did nothing about Lind's suggestions.

Several years later, during Pacific voyages in the 1770s, the famous British explorer James Cook decided to put Lind's theory to the test. During a long voyage, he stocked enough lemon juice to give each crew member a daily ration. It worked. Only one crew member developed scurvy during Cook's exploration.

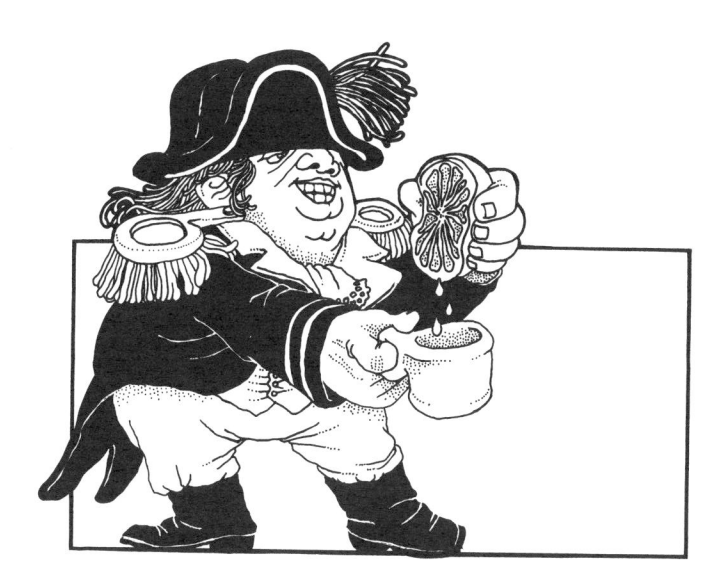

But the Navy refused to change its policies. It was another twenty years before most of the ships carried limes or lime juice, which all sailors were required to consume. And that is how British sailors came to be known as "Limeys."

What Causes Scurvy?

So, citrus fruits cured the disease. But what caused it? The mystery remained unsolved until Casimir Funk, a Polish scientist, began to unravel it in the early 1900s. He was researching a disease called beriberi when he discovered that some substances within fruits, vegetables, and milk are essential to human health. He named those substances "vitamins."

Then, around 1925, a Hungarian scientist named Albert Szent-Gyorgyi isolated a certain type of acid in citrus fruit, and in 1932, a scientist named Charles G. King (along with students at the University of Pittsburgh) analyzed this acid. After running some tests, King and his students realized that the acid was the elusive substance that prevents scurvy. They called the substance ascorbic acid.

We call it vitamin C.

Vitamin A: A Fishy Tale

For many centuries, people have told stories about how certain foods can heal the sick. Some stories have turned out to be "tall tales." Others are grounded in fact. One of the more interesting of these tales led to the discovery of vitamin A.

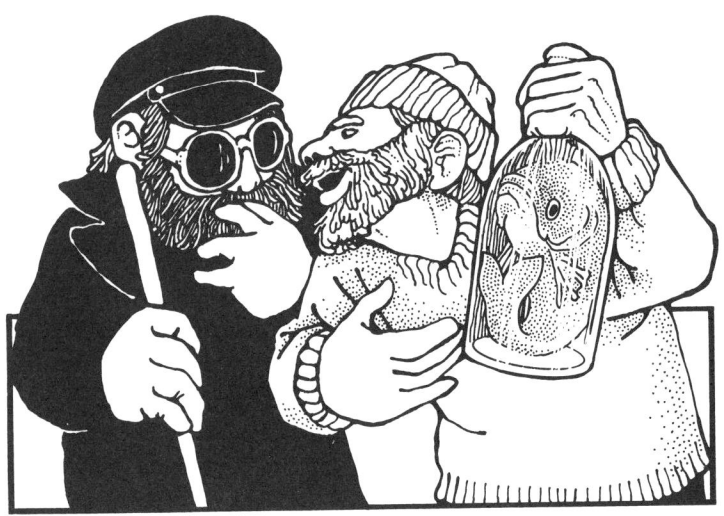

The story starts like this: Long ago, fishermen passed on to their sons and daughters the helpful hint that eating the liver of a fresh fish could cure "night blindness." Night blindness is a condition that keeps people from seeing well in dim light (late in the evening, for example, when the sky is nearly dark). Most people can still see at least a little then. But someone with night blindness can't see at all.

Night blindness was a common problem for fishermen who had been out in the bright sunlight all day long. The fishermen didn't eat much—maybe just some dried bread, cheese, water, and a bit of dried fish. But for some reason, eating a fish liver seemed to solve their sight problem, or so they claimed.

At the time, most scientists thought this idea sounded "fishy" and didn't take it seriously. Then a pair of doctors discovered a substance in eggs and butter that does, in fact, help to repair sunlight-damaged eyes. Later, scientists discovered the same substance in the fatty parts of liver.

Then, in 1912 or so, scientists around the world doing food-related experiments found and isolated this useful stuff and named it vitamin A. People who wanted to maintain good eyesight started taking a spoonful of cod liver oil each day to get their vitamin A.

Three Blind Rats?

Several years later, some scientists were experimenting with laboratory rats that had vitamin A deficiencies. When the rats ate spinach, their vitamin A deficiencies disappeared. Scientists were puzzled by these results, because they knew that spinach does not contain vitamin A. After doing more experiments, they discovered that a substance called carotene was involved. Carotene is a substance that we read and hear a lot about these days.

Carotene is found in leafy green vegetables (like spinach) and yellowish vegetables (like squash and carrots). Carotene does not start out as vitamin A, but our bodies convert it into vitamin A when we eat those vegetables. Substances like carotene that we can convert into vitamins are called "provitamins."

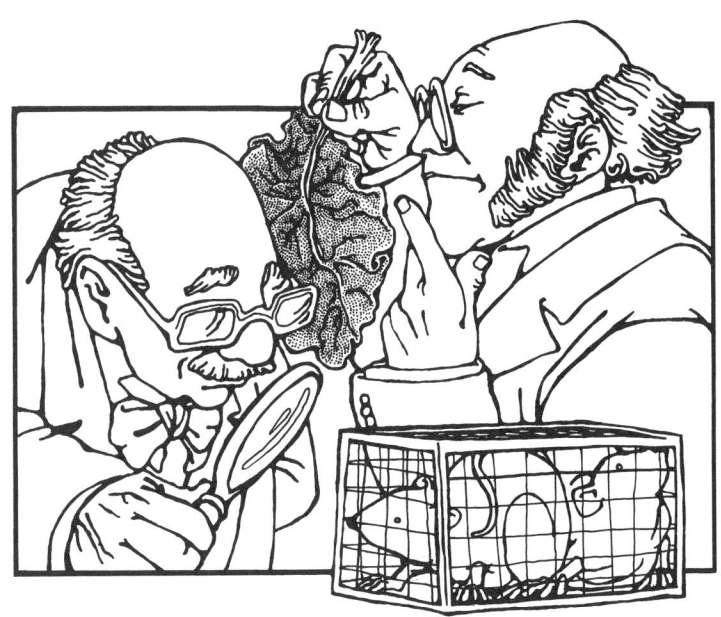

Some nutritionists think that in some ways carotene is the most efficient way for our bodies to get vitamin A. That's because our bodies don't convert carotene into vitamin A until we actually need it, so we don't end up with too much.

The next time someone tells you to eat your spinach or carrots, think about the fishermen of long ago (or the rats—you choose!). You don't have to eat fish liver, but you can eat the right kind of vegetables. Best of all, if you eat vegetables to get your vitamin A, your body will make just the right amount.

Vitamin B-1: The Right Rice

Around 1880, a new disease called beriberi was taking its toll on Japanese sailors. Victims felt very weak, suffered from insomnia, and lost their appetite. Sometimes, their hands and feet became partially paralyzed. Some ships lost a third of their sailors to the disease.

A doctor in the Japanese Navy started to study beriberi. His findings were puzzling. Besides the sailors, rich people in cities (not poor people living in villages) were more likely to get the disease. Also, beriberi occurred most often in countries like Japan, where people ate a lot of rice. British sailors, for example, almost never got the disease.

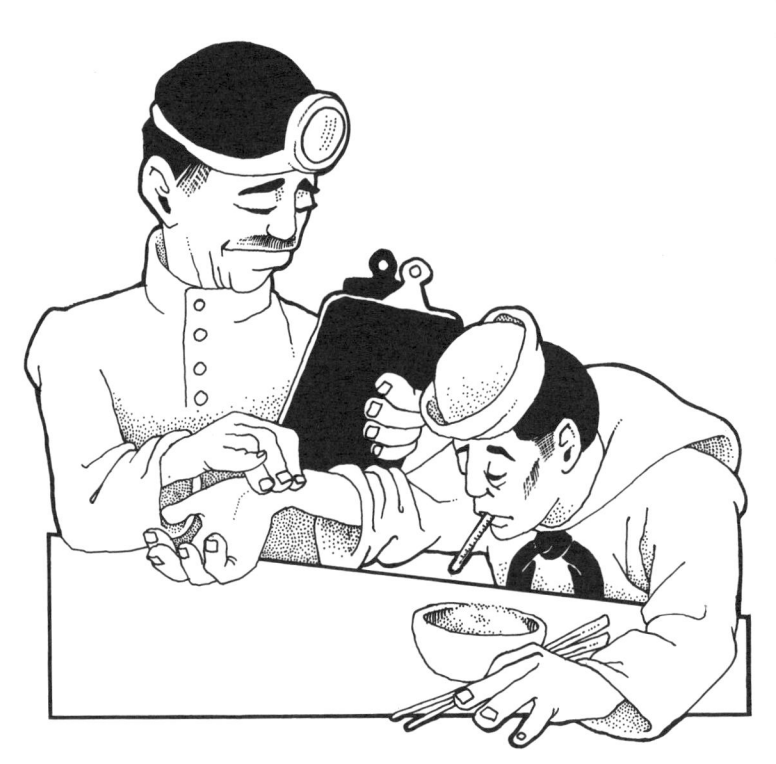

The doctor suspected that diet played a big role in the beriberi problem. How could he test his hypothesis? He decided he would feed Japanese sailors new foods and observe what happened. At first, the Japanese naval officials were insulted; they felt the sailors ate well enough. As they pointed out, the sailors even received the best white rice available, not the cheap brown rice eaten by the villagers. But naval officials also acknowledged that the beriberi had to stop and agreed to allow the experiment.

The doctor noted what happened in 1882 when a Japanese navy ship named the *Riojo* headed for Hawaii via New Zealand and South America. The *Riojo* carried the usual sailor foods—rice and small amounts of vegetables and fish. Within ten months, 169 of the men had contracted beriberi, and 25 had died. The doctor kept careful records of these events.

A year later, the *Tsukua* set sail for the same places as the *Riojo*. But on this journey, the ship carried some other foods as well—oatmeal, canned milk, and extra canned vegetables. Most of the sailors agreed to try the new foods. But 14 of them refused, clinging to their old diets of rice, soups, and small amounts of vegetables and fish. At the end of the journey, those 14 sailors were the only ones who came down with beriberi.

The emperor of Japan was so impressed that he made the doctor a baron. Even more important, he ordered Japanese naval ships to stock more meat, fish, and vegetables and to give at least a pint of milk to each sailor every day. In 1884, the number of beriberi cases among Japanese naval sailors dropped by nearly half. By 1887, instances of beriberi in the Japanese Navy had disappeared.

An Accidental Discovery

Some scientists still had trouble believing that beriberi was related to diet. They thought the disease was caused by a virus or bacteria. But in the early 1900s, American forces fighting in the Philippines stumbled onto a new clue. They took over a Filipino prison, where they found the prisoners eating old, moldy brown rice.

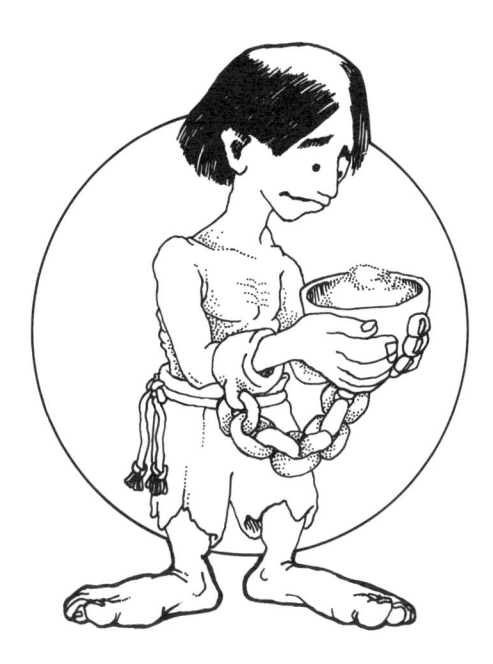

Hoping to improve the poor prisoners' conditions, the Americans started serving polished white rice. Within three months, the number of cases of beriberi in the prison had jumped from 2 to 1,087. The Americans then launched a campaign to sanitize the prison, but that made no difference—the number of cases continued to climb. Finally, a European doctor suggested that the prisoners go back to eating brown rice. Within three months, the number of beriberi cases had dropped to four.

So, why had the Japanese sailors, the wealthy people, and the well-treated prisoners been victims of beriberi? These groups ate mostly processed white rice with the husks of the rice kernels removed. Clearly, there was something in those husks that prevented beriberi. And, apparently, the same substance existed in the food eaten by the Japanese sailors on the *Tsukua* who agreed not to eat rice. But what could this mystery substance be?

In 1906, a team of scientists discovered that when rice husks were soaked in water, the water could cure beriberi. In 1912, Casimir Funk, a Polish chemist, finally isolated the substance that had dissolved into the water. We now call it thiamine, or vitamin B-1.

Today, we add vitamins to white rice to replace those lost during processing. And plain old brown rice—once considered "peasant" food—is starting to make a comeback. As we now know, it is an excellent, natural source of vitamin B-1.

Vitamin D: Shedding Light on Rickets

Next time you eat a peanut butter sandwich and wash it down with a big glass of milk, think about this: both the milk and the peanut butter have first been exposed to ultraviolet light. It may sound like a strange thing to think about, but there is a reason. When ultraviolet light shines on milk and certain oils (like peanut oil), cholesterol is made into vitamin D. And vitamin D helps strengthen bones.

Scientists didn't always know about the value of vitamin D. In fact, it was discovered by accident. A doctor named Alfred Hess was looking for a cure for rickets (a children's bone disease) when he stumbled upon the fact that when you expose certain foods to ultraviolet light, they undergo an unusual reaction. So while seeking the cause of rickets, Hess also discovered its cure—vitamin D.

In the late 1800s, rickets posed a serious threat to children living in cities. The disease caused defective bone growth. And it usually resulted in curved bones and large joints that caused its young victims to walk bowlegged. A child with rickets usually had weak teeth, too.

To find out what caused this horrible disease, Hess fed rats a special diet, free of fats and oils. He and other scientists had already found that this diet caused the rats to develop rickets. But in one case, a group of rats didn't get rickets. Why? These rats had received the same food as the others. So what was different about this group?

The doctor studied everything he could about the rat groups, comparing the ways they ate, slept, and lived. The rats' habits were all the same, except for one seemingly minor detail. The group of healthy rats was kept near an ultraviolet light. Could this be the key to the mystery?

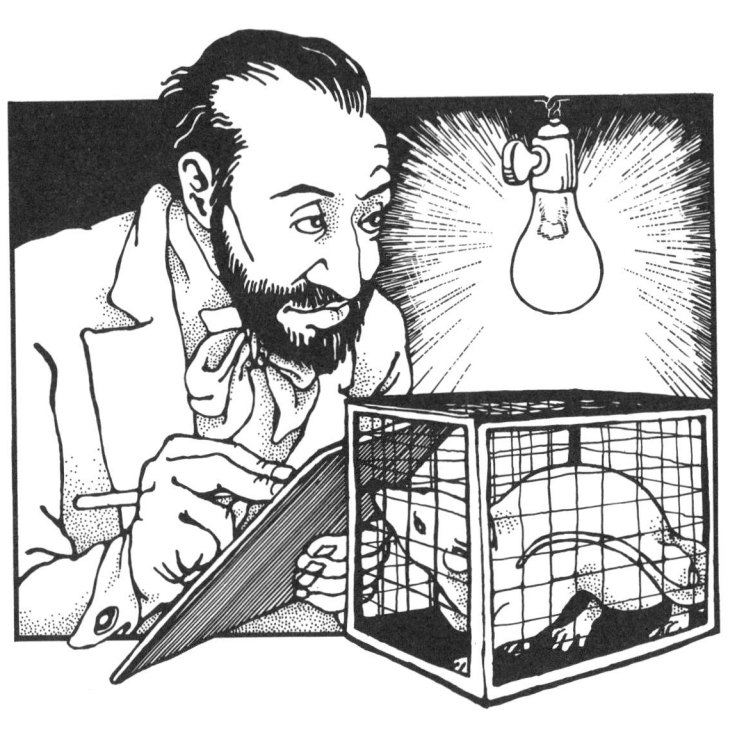

To find out, the doctor set up a new experiment. He formed two new groups of young rats and fed each group the same food. But before feeding Group One, he exposed its food to ultraviolet light. Hess's results were startling: Group One did not develop rickets. The key to preventing this disease was in the light.

Big City Woes

Ultraviolet light also helped explain why rickets was such a problem in the industrialized cities of America and Europe. After the Industrial Revolution, people no longer worked for long hours in sunny fields. Instead, they spent their days laboring in dark factories. More people also moved into cities, which became crowded.

And children were often raised in cramped urban conditions and sent off to work at a young age. All of this, combined with long, dark, winter months, greatly decreased the amount of light present in people's lives. And it greatly increased the number of children with rickets.

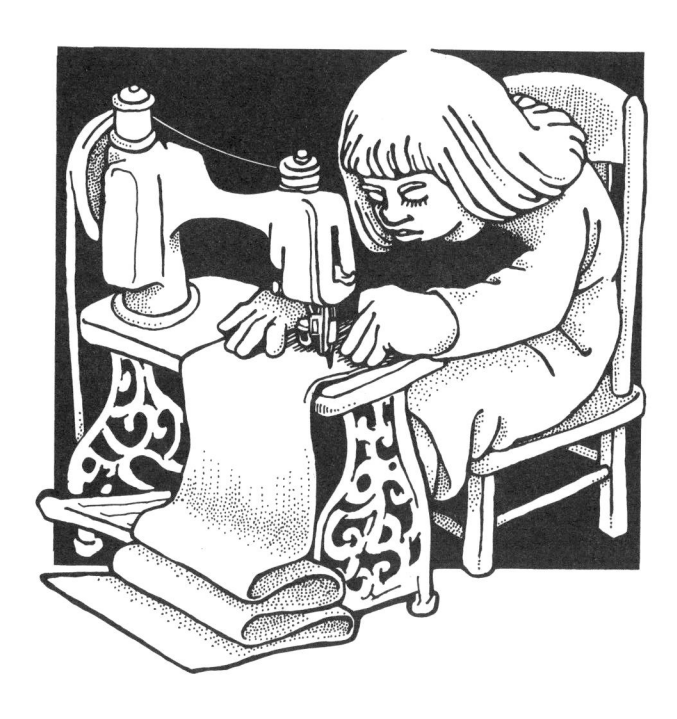

Until Hess's experiments, people had debated for years about the true cause of rickets. Some folks thought it was contagious, like measles or chicken pox. Others thought it could be cured by a dose of cod liver oil. Then Hess "shed some light" on the subject. But he still wasn't sure why ultraviolet light made such a difference.

The question of "why" was answered in the 1920s. Scientists found a way to isolate the new substance that is created (in food and in our bodies) when ultraviolet light shines on the cholesterol in fats and oils. Eventually, this substance was named vitamin D.

But what does vitamin D have to do with bones? Well, it turns out that vitamin D plays a role in the way our bodies absorb calcium—a key part of bones. Without vitamin D, our bones can't be strong. Isn't it lucky for us that Hess made the connection between ultraviolet light and rickets? Now we can make sure we eat foods with plenty of vitamin D.

Blackline Master

VITAMIN FORTIFIED
CORN FLAKES

INGREDIENTS:
MILLED YELLOW CORN, SUGAR, SALT, MALT SYRUP, CORN SYRUP.

VITAMINS AND MINERALS:
SODIUM ASCORBATE (VITAMIN C), NIACINAMIDE, REDUCED IRON, PYRIDOXINE HYDROCHLORIDE (VITAMIN B_6), VITAMIN A PALMITATE, RIBOFLAVIN (VITAMIN B_2), THIAMINE MONONITRATE (VITAMIN B_1), FOLIC ACID, AND VITAMIN D.

BHT ADDED TO PACKAGING MATERIAL TO HELP PRESERVE FRESHNESS.

NUTRITION INFORMATION PER SERVING

SERVING SIZE 1 OZ. (1 CUP)
SERVINGS PER CONTAINER 18

	1 OZ. CORN FLAKES	WITH ½ CUP VITAMINS A & D FORTIFIED SKIM MILK
CALORIES	110	150*
PROTEIN	2 g	6 g
CARBOHYDRATE	25 g	31 g
FAT	0 g	0 g*
CHOLESTEROL	0 mg	0 mg*
SODIUM	270 mg	330 mg
POTASSIUM	25 mg	230 mg

PERCENTAGE OF U.S. RECOMMENDED DAILY ALLOWANCES (U.S. RDA)

PROTEIN	2	10
VITAMIN A	25	30
VITAMIN C	25	25
THIAMINE	25	30
RIBOFLAVIN	25	35
NIACIN	25	25
CALCIUM	**	15
IRON	10	10
VITAMIN D	10	25
VITAMIN B_6	25	25
FOLIC ACID	25	25

*CEREAL PLUS ½ CUP WHOLE MILK CONTAINS 180 CALORIES, 4 g FAT AND 15 mg CHOLESTEROL.
**CONTAINS LESS THAN 2 PERCENT OF THE U.S. RDA OF THIS NUTRIENT.

CARBOHYDRATE INFORMATION

	1 OZ. CORN FLAKES	WITH MILK
STARCH AND RELATED CARBOHYDRATES	22 g	22 g
SUCROSE AND OTHER SUGARS	2 g	8 g
DIETARY FIBER	1 g	1 g
TOTAL CARBOHYDRATES	25 g	31 g

VALUES BY FORMULATION AND ANALYSIS

STC / *Food Chemistry*

Blackline Master

INSTANT RICE

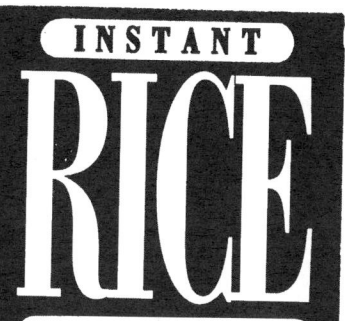

NUTRITION INFORMATION PER SERVING

Serving size......1 oz.
(About ½ cup prepared)
Servings
  per container.....28
Calories...........110
Protein.............2g
Carbohydrate......23g
Fat................0g
Sodium..........0mg
(As packaged)

PERCENTAGE OF U.S. RECOMMENDED DAILY ALLOWANCES (U.S. RDA)

Protein.............2
Vitamin A...........*
Vitamin C...........*
Thiamine............8
Riboflavin..........*
Niacin..............6
Calcium.............*
Iron................4

*Contains less than 2% of the U.S. RDA of these nutrients.

Ingredients: Precooked long grain rice enriched with niacin (niacinamide), iron (ferric orthophosphate), thiamine (thiamine hydrochloride).

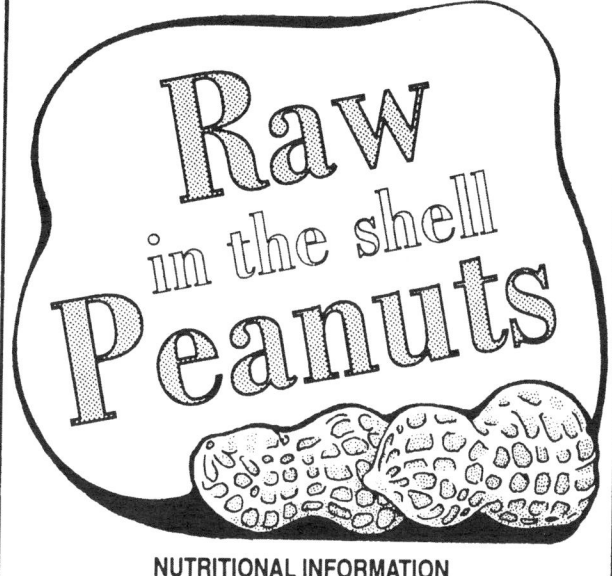

Raw in the shell Peanuts

NUTRITIONAL INFORMATION

Serving	100 grams/3.2 oz. Shelled Weight	Iron (mg)	2.1
Calories	564	Sodium (mg)	5
Protein (grams)	26	Potassium (mg)	674
Water	5.6%	Vitamin A (IU)	*
Fat (grams)	47.5	Thiamin (mg)	1.14
Carbohydrates (grams)	18.6	Riboflavin (mg)	.13
Fiber (grams)	2.4	Niacin (mg)	17.2
Phosphorus (mg)	401	Ascorbic Acid (mg)	*

*Contains less than 2% of the US RDA of these nutrients. Source: USDA Handbook.

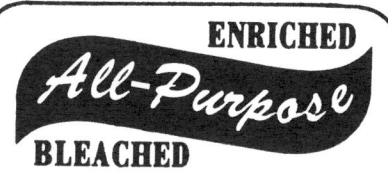

ENRICHED All-Purpose BLEACHED FLOUR

INGREDIENTS: BLEACHED WHEAT FLOUR, BARLEY MALT FLOUR, NIACIN, IRON, THIAMINE, MONONITRATE, RIBOFLAVIN.

NUTRITION INFORMATION PER SERVING

SERVING SIZE.....1 CUP (APPROX 4 OZ)
SERVINGS PER CONTAINER...........8
CALORIES........................400
PROTEIN.........................11 g
CARBOHYDRATE....................87 g
FAT.............................1 g
SODIUM..........................0 mg

PERCENTAGE OF U.S. RECOMMENDED DAILY ALLOWANCES (U.S. RDA)

PROTEIN.........................15
VITAMIN A........................*
VITAMIN C........................*
THIAMINE........................45
RIBOFLAVIN......................25
NIACIN..........................30
CALCIUM..........................2
IRON............................20
PHOSPHORUS......................10

*CONTAINS LESS THAN 2% OF THE U.S. RDA OF THESE NUTRIENTS.

ALL NATURAL NO PRESERVATIVES

Honey-Oats GRANOLA BARS

NUTRITION INFORMATION PER SERVING

SERVING SIZE..............1 bar
SERVINGS PER CONTAINER.....12
CALORIES..................110
PROTEIN....................2g
CARBOHYDRATE..............16g
FAT........................4g
SODIUM...................65mg

PERCENTAGE OF U.S. RECOMMENDED DAILY ALLOWANCES (U.S. RDA)

PROTEIN.....................4
VITAMIN A...................*
VITAMIN C...................*
THIAMINE....................4
RIBOFLAVIN..................*
NIACIN......................*
CALCIUM.....................*
IRON........................*

*CONTAINS LESS THAN 2% OF THE U.S. RDA OF THESE NUTRIENTS

INGREDIENTS: ROLLED OATS, BROWN SUGAR, SUNFLOWER OIL, HONEY, SALT, LECITHIN, NATURAL VANILLA.

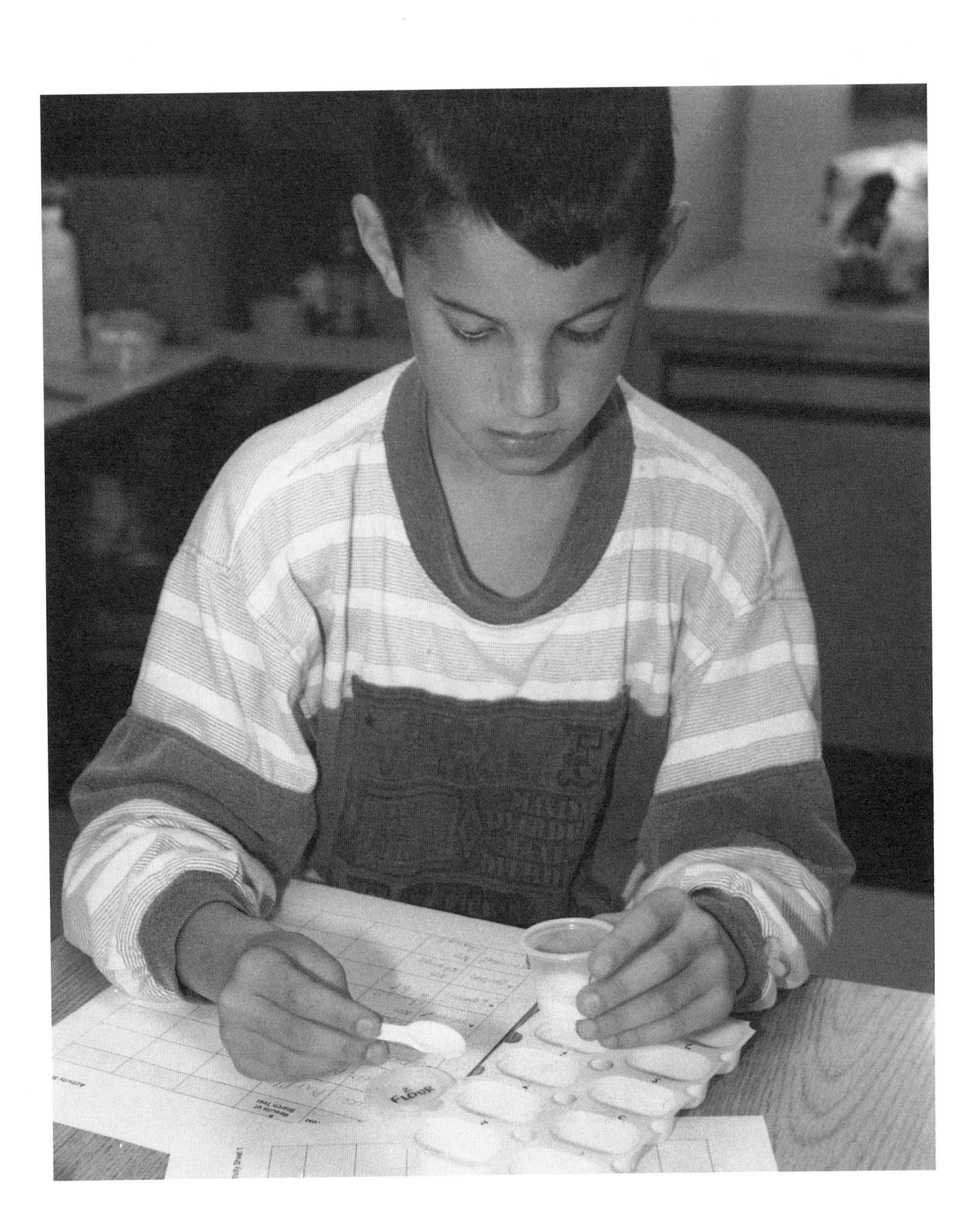

LESSON 16

What Is in a Marshmallow? Applying What We Have Learned

Overview and Objectives

This lesson challenges students to apply what they have learned about testing foods as they test a new food—a marshmallow. Students also demonstrate their ability to interpret food labels, make comparisons between label information and test results, and judge why a food might or might not be a good nutritional choice in a given situation. These activities offer you useful information with which to assess student progress.

- Students predict which nutrients—starch, glucose, fats, and proteins—they think are present in a marshmallow.

- Students design a test table for recording the results of four nutrient tests on a marshmallow.

- Students apply the tests learned in the unit to the marshmallow and compare their test results with information found on a marshmallow package label.

- Students record their findings about the nutritional content of the marshmallow in their notebooks and share in a class discussion about healthy foods.

Background

When students test the marshmallow, they may be surprised to discover that it actually does contain many of the nutrients they know how to test for. Figure 16-1 shows one example of a test table (your students may come up with other formats) and typical test results.

Later, when students look at the ingredients on a marshmallow package label, they may also be surprised to find that the marshmallow contains corn syrup, water, and cornstarch. And they may recognize corn syrup as the liquid that tested positive for glucose, and cornstarch as the liquid that tested positive for starch.

Materials

For each student
    1 science notebook
    1 marshmallow label

For every two students
    1 marshsmallow

STC / *Food Chemistry*

LESSON 16

Figure 16-1

Sample table and test results

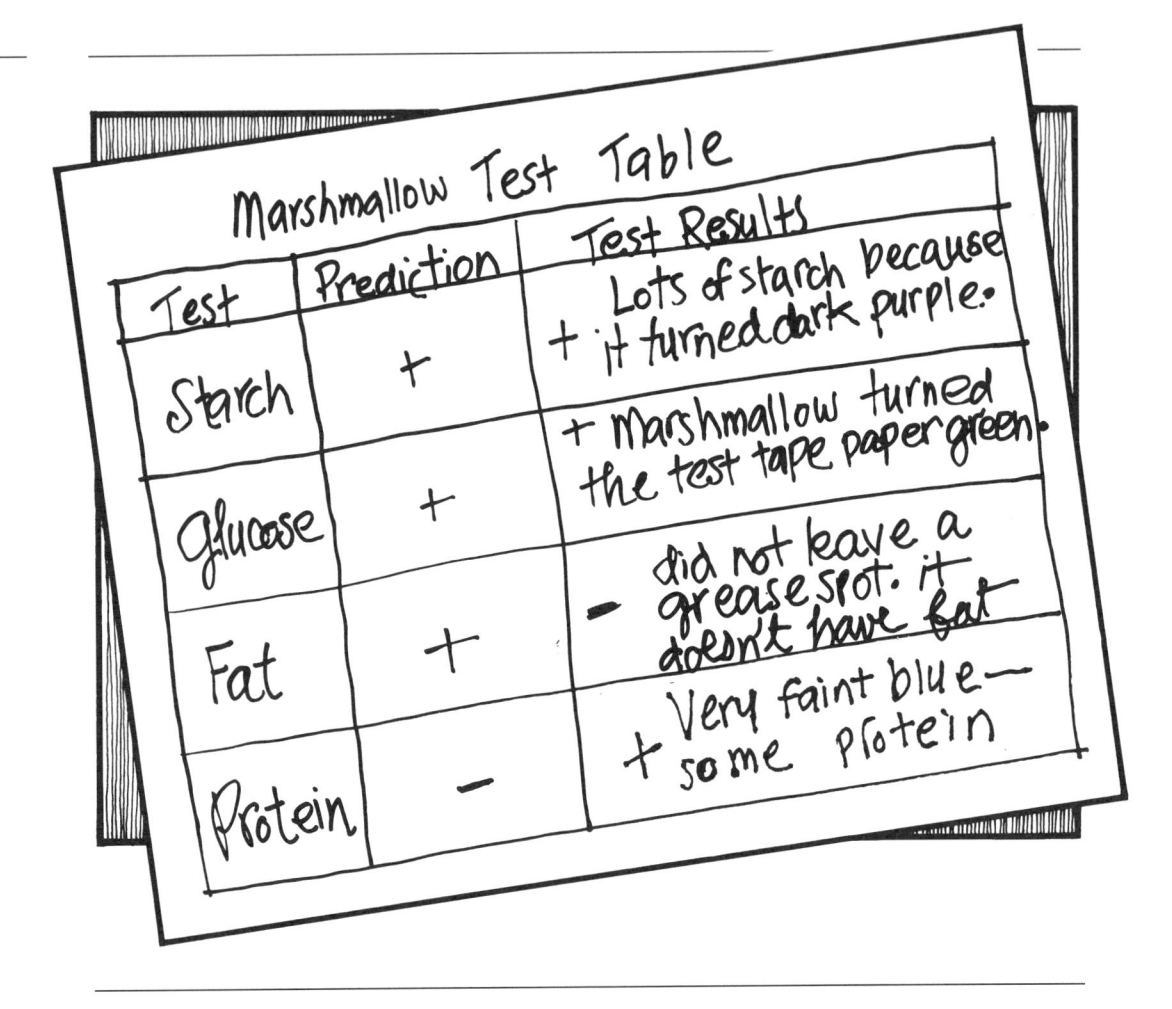

Marshmallow Test Table

Test	Prediction	Test Results
Starch	+	+ Lots of starch because it turned dark purple.
Glucose	+	+ marshmallow turned the test tape paper green.
Fat	+	– did not leave a grease spot. It doesn't have fat
Protein	–	+ Very faint blue — some protein

For every four students
- 1 storage bag containing the following:
  - 1 food bag
  - 2 lab bags
  - 1 liquids bag
- 2 strips of glucose test paper
- 2 strips of Coomassie blue test paper
- 1 petri dish
- 2 pieces of brown paper, approximately 5 cm x 10 cm (2" x 4")
- Toothpicks

For the class
- Developing solution (white vinegar and rubbing alcohol)
- Cleanup materials (2 plastic-lined disposal boxes, sponges, paper towels)
- Soapy water (sink or buckets)
- Clear water (sink or buckets)

LESSON 16

Figure 16-2

What is in a marshmallow?

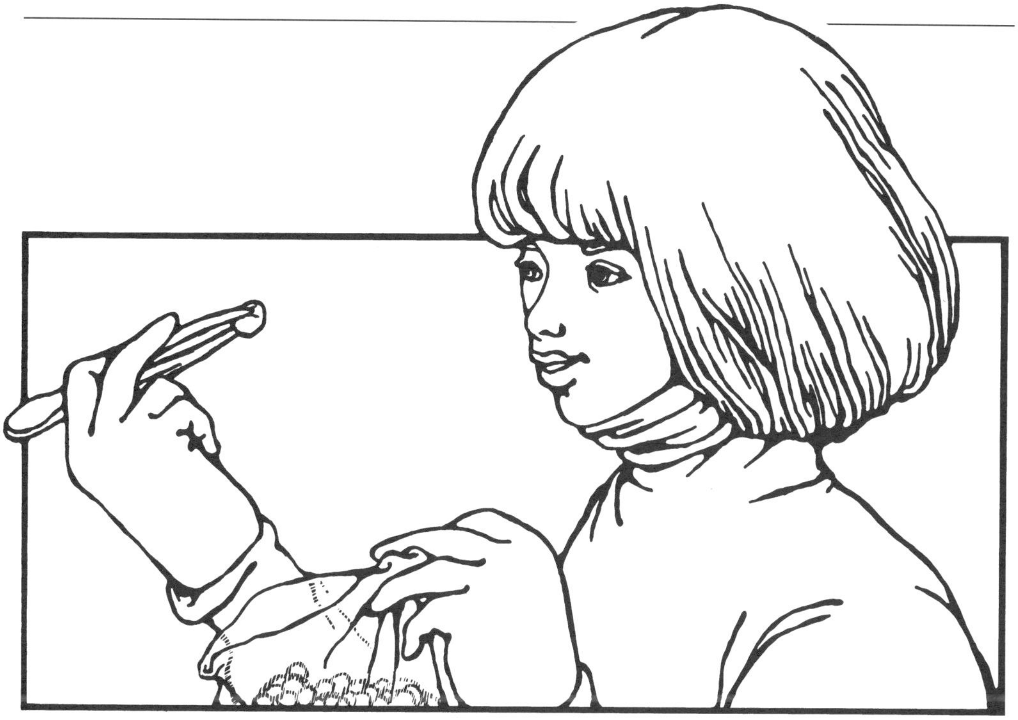

Preparation

1. Have students help you prepare all the materials used in the starch, glucose, fats, and proteins tests.

2. Copy one marshmallow label for each student by xeroxing the blackline master on pg. 166.

Procedure

1. Ask students which nutrients they think are in a marshmallow and why. Explain that today they will test a marshmallow for starch, glucose, fats, and proteins.

2. As a class, briefly review each of the four chemical tests. Encourage students to refer back to their notebooks, tables, or Student Activity Books to help them remember the procedures.

3. Tell students that, once again, they will create a table to record their data. Point out to students that today's table will look different from previous ones since they will test only one food—the marshmallow—but perform all four tests.

4. Before students draw the tables, have them discuss with their groups how the tables might look and what information should be included. After students have drawn the tables, have them record their predictions.

5. Now, have one student from each group of four pick up the materials needed for all four tests and let students get to work. As before, you will need to pour the protein test developing solution into the petri dishes.

6. After students have performed the tests, recorded results, and cleaned up, ask them to write a few sentences in their notebooks about whether marshmallows would be a good snack for a long hike. Ask students to include at least two reasons supporting their opinions.

LESSON 16

7. Then ask the class to share what they found out by discussing the following questions:

   - How did your results compare with your predictions?
   - Which nutrients are present in the marshmallow?
   - What additional information might be found on a marshmallow package label?

Management Tip: Since this is a long lesson, you may want to do the **Final Activities** during another period.

Final Activities

1. Tell students that they are going to compare their test results with the information on a marshmallow label. Have each student construct a new table on which to record this data.

2. Next, distribute one marshmallow label to each student. Ask students to compare their test results with the information on the label and to complete the table.

3. Have a class discussion to share results. The following questions may be helpful:

   - Did your test results and the label agree?
   - List the marshmallow's nutrients in order from most present to least present. How do you know?
   - What are the ingredients in a marshmallow? What do you already know about some of these ingredients?

4. Finally, ask students if their opinion has changed about whether marshmallows are a good choice for a snack on a long hike. After a brief discussion, have students explain in their notebooks why their opinion has or has not changed.

Extensions

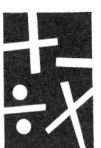

1. Have students describe in writing how they think marshmallows are made. Then, have the class write a letter to a marshmallow manufacturer and ask for an explanation of how marshmallows actually are made.

2. How do marshmallows compare nutritionally with other snack foods, such as candy bars and packaged cookies? Have students research several snack foods and make a graph comparing nutritional contents.

Assessments

This lesson offers you several opportunities to assess students' current ability to apply tests, interpret information, and relate that information to aspects of nutrition. Consider the following criteria when you are assessing your students' learning.

Lab Procedures

- Did students correctly follow the procedures for each test?
- Did students avoid contaminating materials?

Discussions
- Can students describe the tests they conducted?
- Can students identify the nutrients in a marshmallow?
- Can students describe how their test results compared with the marshmallow label?
- Can students name information, other than nutrient values, that appears on food labels?
- Can students identify the ingredients in a marshmallow?
- Do students recognize that corn syrup is the main ingredient in a marshmallow? Can they connect this realization to what they know about glucose?

Written Work
- Did students construct a test table that included predictions, test results, and conclusions (such as "lots of starch," or "some protein," as in Figure 16-1)?
- Did students record complete, legible data on their test table?
- Did students include at least two reasons why they think marshmallows are or are not a good choice for a long hike?
- Did students include the ingredients on the table they constructed to compare test results with the label?
- In the **Final Activities**, did students clearly explain why they did or did not change their opinion about taking marshmallows as a snack on a long hike?

Post-Unit Assessment

The post-unit assessment on pg. 169 is a matched follow-up to the pre-unit assessment in Lesson 1. By comparing students' pre- and post-unit responses, you will be able to document their growth in knowledge about nutrients contained in foods.

Final Assessments

Final assessments for this unit are provided in **Appendix A**, on pg. 171. They include a self-assessment for students and assessments on applying nutrient tests and interpreting food labels.

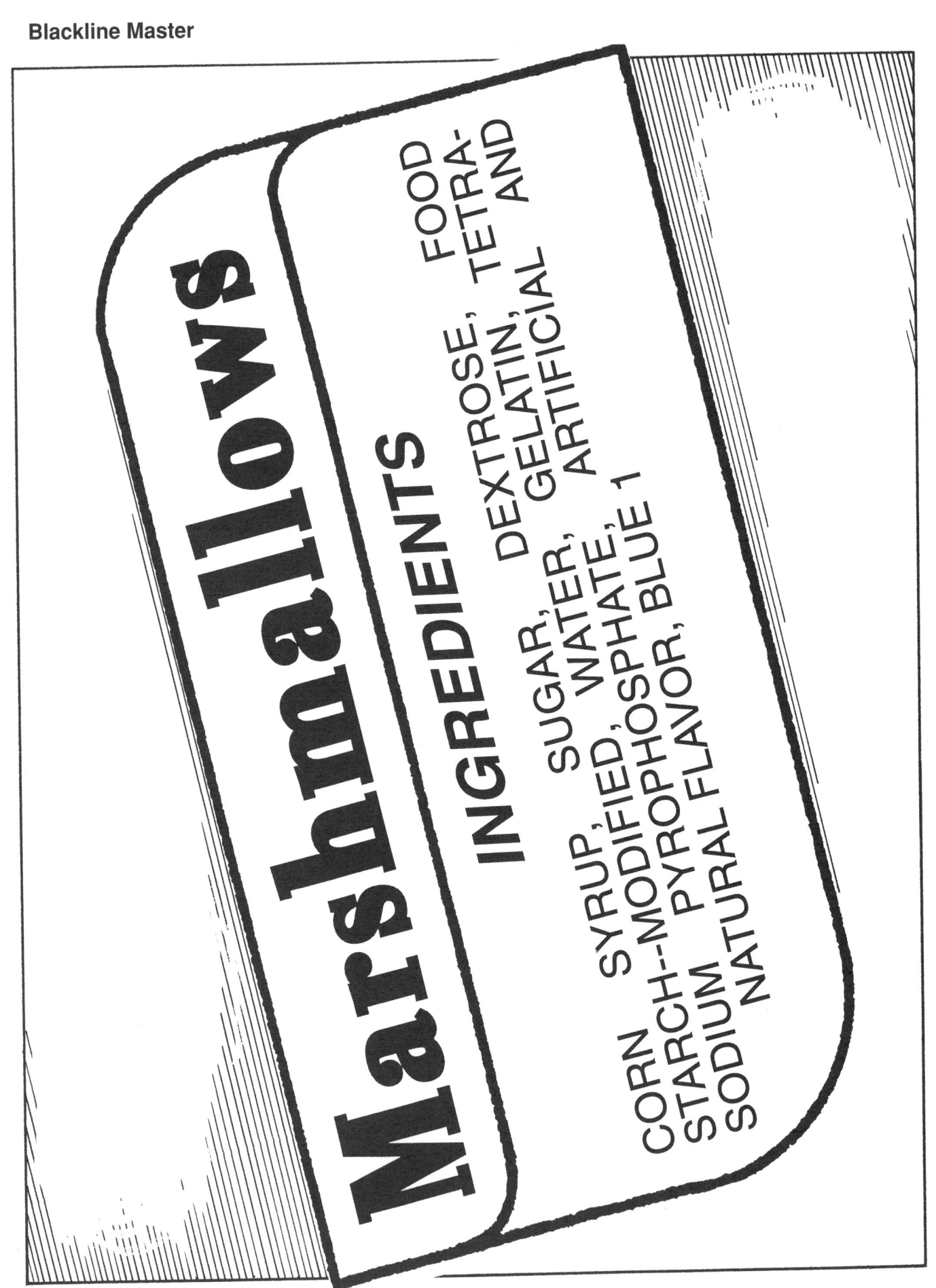

Marshmallows

INGREDIENTS: CORN SYRUP, SUGAR, DEXTROSE, WATER, GELATIN, MODIFIED STARCH, SODIUM TETRA-PYROPHOSPHATE, ARTIFICIAL AND NATURAL FLAVOR, BLUE 1 FOOD

Post-Unit Assessment

Overview

This is the second part of the matched pre- and post-unit assessments of students' ideas about the foods they eat. By comparing the individual and class responses from Lesson 1 with those from this activity, you will be able to document students' learning over the course of the unit. During the first brainstorming session, students developed two lists—"What We Know about Foods" and "Questions We Have about Foods"—as well as a Venn diagram of foods eaten for different meals. When they revisit these during the assessment, students may realize how much they have learned about foods, nutrients, and conducting chemical tests.

Materials

For each student
- 1 science notebook
- 1 blank sheet of unlined paper

For the class
- Two class lists and the Venn diagram from Lesson 1

Procedure

1. Ask students to review their notebooks and record charts. What do they now know about the foods they eat? What questions do they now have? Ask them to spend a few minutes writing their thoughts in their notebooks. When you compare students' notebook entries from Lesson 1 with their entries in this matched post-unit assessment, look for both refinement of ideas and evidence given in support of ideas.

2. Display the two class lists from Lesson 1—"What We Know about Foods" and "Questions We Have about Foods." Ask students to identify statements that they now know to be true. What experiences did they have during the unit that confirmed these statements? Then ask students to identify statements they would like to correct or improve. Again, they should support their conclusions with evidence or experiences from the unit.

3. Now ask students to share their notebook entries about the new information they learned during this unit. Add their statements to the "What We Know about Foods" list.

Post-Unit Assessment

4. Ask students to share the new questions they have about foods. Add their questions to the "Questions We Have about Foods" list.

5. Have students review the Venn diagram from Lesson 1. Challenge them to think of another way to categorize foods. Distribute blank sheets of paper. Ask students to create a Venn diagram that uses the presence of nutrients as a way to categorize the foods they eat.

APPENDIX A	**Final Assessments**

Overview

Following are some suggestions for assessment activities. Although it is not essential to do all these activities, it is recommended that students do Assessment 1.

- Assessment 1 is a questionnaire that students can use to evaluate themselves.

- Assessment 2 asks students to identify mystery foods by repeating the foods tests.

- Assessment 3 asks students to read and interpret some actual food labels.

Assessment 1

Student Self-Assessment

Using a questionnaire, students assess their own learning and participation during the unit.

Materials

For each student
1   Student Self-Assessment (on pg. 172)

Procedure

1. Distribute a copy of the Student Self-Assessment to each student and then preview it with the class. Explain to the students that it is important to stop from time to time and think about how they are working.

2. Allow students sufficient time to complete the self-assessment either in class or as a homework assignment.

STC / *Food Chemistry*

Food Chemistry:
Student Self-Assessment

Name: _____

Date: _____

1. What have you learned from doing the activities in the *Food Chemistry* unit that you think is important?

2. How well do you think you and your partner(s) worked together? Give some examples.

3. Identify the activities in the unit that you particularly enjoyed. Explain why you liked them.

4. Were there any activities in the unit that you did not understand or that confused you? Explain your answer.

5. Take another look at your Record Sheets and your science notebook. Describe how well you think you recorded your observations and ideas.

6. How do you feel about science? (Circle the words that apply to you.)
    a. Interested
    b. Bored
    c. Nervous
    d. Excited
    e. Confused
    f. Successful
    g. Write down one word of your own _____

APPENDIX A

Assessment 2 — Identifying Mystery Foods

Students apply test procedures established for starch, glucose, fats, and proteins. They should review the information about these tests in their science notebooks before testing this new food.

Materials

For each student
- 1 science notebook

For every two students
- 1 "mystery" food (use a food that is a common snack or lunch-box item for your students, but crumble or dissolve it in a small amount of water so that it is not easily recognized)
- 1 plastic storage bag containing the following:
  - 1 lab bag
  - 1 set of test materials

Procedure

1. Distribute the mystery food to students. Ask students to write their ideas about the food in their notebooks.
2. Ask students to plan their tests to determine the nutrients in the food. Also have them prepare a record sheet for the tests.
3. Distribute the plastic bag containing the lab bag and test materials. Have students test the food.
4. Ask students to complete the record sheet and then, in their notebooks, write what they now know about the food.

Assessment 3 — Interpreting Food Labels

Applying their experiences with the nutrient tests and food labels, students describe the nutrients found in unidentified foods. Students also describe how each food would be part of a "healthy" diet.

Materials

For each student
- 1 science notebook
- 1 copy of **Figure A-1, Sample Food Labels**

Procedure

1. Reproduce the sample labels in Figure A-1 and give one copy to each student. For your information only, Label A is from Froot Loops™ cereal, Label B is from peanut butter, and Label C is from Hooplas™ crunchy corn chips.
2. Ask students to read each label and, in their science notebooks, write anything they think they can say about the nutrients and vitamins in this food.
3. Ask students to write in their science notebooks about when and why they might eat each food.
4. Reveal the identities of the foods after students have written their thoughts about the labels.

APPENDIX A

Figure A-1

Sample Food Labels

Label A
NUTRITION INFORMATION

Serving Size: 1 oz (28.4 g, about 1 cup)
Servings per Package: 15

Per Serving:
Calories	110
Protein	2 g
Carbohydrate	25 g
Fat, Total	1 g
Unsaturated	1 g
Saturated	0 g
Cholesterol	0 g
Sodium	125 mg
Potassium	30 mg

Percentage of U.S. Recommended Daily Allowances (U.S. RDA)

Protein	2
Vitamin A	15
Vitamin C	100
Thiamin	25
Riboflavin	25
Niacin	25
Calcium	*
Iron	25
Vitamin D	10
Vitamin B_6	25
Folic Acid	25
Phosphorus	2
Magnesium	2
Zinc	25
Copper	2

*Contains less than 2% of the U.S. RDA of this nutrient.

Ingredients: Corn, Wheat, and Oat Flour; Sugar; Partially Hydrogenated Vegetable Oil; Salt, Yellow #6, Turmeric Color; Red #40; Natural Orange, Lemon, and Cherry and Other Natural Flavorings; Blue #1;

Vitamins and Minerals: Vitamin C (Sodium Ascorbate and Ascorbic Acid); Niacinamide; Zinc (Oxide): Iron; Vitamin B_6 (Pyridoxine Hydrochloride): Vitamin B_2 (Riboflavin); Vitamin A; Vitamin B_1 (Thiamin Hydrochloride); Folic Acid; and Vitamin D.

Label B
NUTRITION INFORMATION

Serving Size: 2 tblsps. (32 g)
Servings per Container: 15

Per Serving:
Calories	190
Protein	9 g
Carbohydrate	6 g
Fat	16 g
% of Calories from Fat	73
Polyunsaturated	5 g
Saturated	3 g
Cholesterol (0 mg/100g)	0 mg
Sodium	150 mg

Percentage of U. S. Recommended Daily Allowance (U.S. RDA)

Protein	15
Vitamin A	*
Vitamin C	*
Thiamine	*
Riboflavin	*
Niacin	20
Calcium	*
Iron	2

*Contains less than 2% of the U.S. RDA of these nutrients.

Ingredients: Peanuts and Salt

Label C
NUTRITION INFORMATION

Serving Size: 1 oz
Servings per Container: 8

Per Serving:
Calories	140
Protein	2 g
Carbohydrate	17 g
Fat	8 g
Polyunsaturated	4 g
Saturated	1 g
Cholesterol	0 mg
Sodium	240 mg
Potassium	55 mg

Percentage of the U. S. Recommended Daily Allowance (U.S. RDA)

Protein	2
Vitamin A	*
Vitamin C	*
Thiamine	2
Riboflavin	2
Niacin	2
Calcium	4
Iron	2

*Contains less than 2% of the U.S. RDA of this nutrient.

Ingredients: Corn, Vegetable Oil (Corn Oil and Partially Hydrogenated Cottonseed and Soybean Oils with THBQ to Preserve Freshness), Modified Food Starch, Salt, Dehydrated Cheddar, Romano and Parmesan Cheeses, (Pasteurized Milk, Cheese Cultures, Salt, Enzymes), Whey, Dehydrated Tomato, Monosodium Glutamate, Dehydrated Onion & Garlic, Maltodextrin, Mono- & Diglycerides, Artificial Colors, Buttermilk, Dehydrated Cream, Disodium Phosphate, Disodium Inosinate and Disodium Guanylate, Extractives of Annatto, Paprika and Turmeric, Citric Acid, Spice.

APPENDIX B

Bibliography

The **Bibliography** is divided into the following categories:

- Resources for Teachers
- Resources for Students

While not a complete list of the many books written on food chemistry and nutrition, this is a sampling of books that complement this unit. These materials come well recommended. They have been favorably reviewed, and teachers have found them useful.

If a book goes out of print or if you seek additional titles, you may wish to consult the following resources.

Appraisal: Science Books for Young People (The Children's Science Book Review Committee, Boston, MA).

> Published quarterly, this periodical reviews new science books available for young people. Each book is reviewed by a librarian and by a scientist. The Children's Science Book Review Committee is sponsored by the Science Education Department of Boston University's School of Education and the New England Roundtable of Children's Librarians.

National Science Resources Center. *Science for Children: Resources for Teachers.* Washington, DC: National Academy Press, 1988.

> This volume provides a wealth of information about resources for hands-on science programs. It reviews science curriculum materials, supplementary materials (science activity books, books on teaching science, reference books, and magazines), museum programs, and elementary science curriculum projects.

Science and Children (National Science Teachers Association, Washington, DC).

> Each March, this monthly periodical includes an annotated bibliography of outstanding children's science trade books primarily for pre-kindergarten through eighth-grade science teachers.

Science Books & Films (American Association for the Advancement of Science, Washington, DC).

> Published nine times a year, this periodical offers critical reviews of a wide range of science materials, from books to audiovisual materials to electronic resources. The reviews are primarily written by scientists and science educators. *Science Books & Films* is useful for librarians, media specialists, curriculum supervisors, science teachers, and others responsible for recommending and purchasing scientific materials.

Scientific American (Scientific American, Inc., New York).

> Each December, Philip and Phylis Morrison compile and review a selection of outstanding new science books for children.

Sosa, Maria, and Shirley M. Malcom, eds. *Science Books & Films: Best Books for Children, 1988-91.* Washington, DC: American Association for the Advancement of Science Press, 1992.

> This volume, part of a continuing series, is a compilation of the most highly rated science books that have been reviewed recently in the periodical *Science Books & Film*.

Resources for Teachers

Dishon, Dee, and Pat Wilson O'Leary. *A Guidebook for Cooperative Learning: Techniques for Creating More Effective Schools.* Holmes Beach, FL: Learning Publications, Inc., 1984.

> A practical guide to help teachers implement cooperative learning in the classroom.

Food and Nutrition Board, Institute of Medicine. *Improving America's Diet and Health: From Recommendations to Action.* Edited by Paul R. Thomas. Washington, DC: National Academy Press, 1991.

> Explores how various factors influence our diet, why previous dietary programs have failed, and how Americans can be persuaded to adopt healthier eating habits.

Johnson, David W., Roger T. Johnson, and Edythe Johnson Holubec. *Circles of Learning: Cooperation in the Classroom.* Alexandria, VA: Association for Supervision and Curriculum Development, 1984.

> Presents the case for cooperative learning in a concise and readable form. Reviews the research, outlines implementation strategies, and answers many questions.

McGee, Harold. *On Food and Cooking: The Science and Lore of the Kitchen.* New York: Macmillan, 1988.

> Includes much information relating to chemistry, nutrition, culture, history, geography, and health. Thorough and appropriate for those with little or no background in science.

Resources for Students

Alvarado, Manuel. *Mexican Food and Drink.* New York: Bookwright Press, 1988.

>Introduces students to Mexican culture and geography. Helps children see that plants and animals provide different foods in the Mexican diet and also shows the occupations involved in food processing.

Asimov, Isaac. *How Did We Find Out about Vitamins?* New York: Walker and Company, 1974.

>A historical account of the discovery of vitamins. Introduces the different scientists who played an important role in the discovery of these vitamins.

Burns, Marilyn. *Good for Me!* Boston: Little Brown and Company, 1978.

>Introduces children to what eating is and why it is important. Provides activities and opportunities to do further investigations.

Cobb, Vicki. *Gobs of Goo.* New York: J. B. Lippincott, 1983.

>Describes various types of sticky substances and shows how they are used in everyday life. The topics in the book correlate strongly with the lessons in *Food Chemistry*.

Downer, Lesley. *Japanese Food and Drink.* New York: Bookwright Press, 1988.

>Provides a cultural background to important foods in the Japanese diet.

Gibbons, Gail. *The Milk Makers.* New York: Macmillan Publishing Company, 1985.

>Explains how cows produce milk and how it is processed before being delivered to stores. Aimed at the younger reader, with illustrations on each page and brief text.

Miller, Judy. *Grilled Cheese at Four O'Clock in the Morning.* Washington, DC: American Diabetes Association, 1988.

>Helps students understand what it is like to be a child with diabetes and explains the kinds of everyday adjustments diabetics make to cope with the disease.

Mitchell, Barbara. *A Pocketful of Goobers: A Story about George Washington Carver.* Minneapolis: Carolrhoda Books, 1986.

>Details George Washington Carver's contributions, as a scientist and chemist, to the food industry.

Mitgutsch, Ali. *From Beet to Sugar.* Minneapolis: Carolrhoda Books, 1972; *From Cacao Bean to Chocolate.* Minneapolis: Carolrhoda Books, 1975.

>Short accounts of how sugar is processed and how chocolate is made.

Osborne, Christine. *Southeast Asian Food and Drink.* New York: Bookwright Press, 1989.

>Gives children background information about important foods in the Asian diet, where these foods grow, and how they are processed.

APPENDIX B

Rice, Karen. *Does Candy Grow on Trees?* New York: Walker and Company, 1984.

> Details the origins of different ingredients in candies and sweet foods. Also portrays how different plants play an important role in different foods.

Roberts, Willo Davis. *Sugar Isn't Everything.* New York: Macmillan, 1988.

> A short novel about a girl with diabetes and how she copes with her disease.

Showers, Paul. *What Happens to a Hamburger?* New York: Harper and Row, 1985.

> A brief account of digestion and why it is important to eat a variety of foods.

Ward, Brian R. *Diet and Nutrition.* New York: Franklin Watts, 1987.

> Covers nutrition and its role in health. Provides an excellent introduction to each nutrient and why nutrients are important. Also discusses different ways to organize foods.

APPENDIX C

Making Test Solutions and Papers

Making Starch Test Solution
The iodine solution used to test for starch may be purchased from Carolina Biological Supply Company. Alternatively, you can make your own solution.

To make the solution yourself

1. Iodine may be purchased from a pharmacy. The "tincture of iodine" sold in the pharmacy is typically a 4.4% solution, which should be diluted for use as a starch indicator. Do not purchase the iodine labeled "decolorized"; it will not work as a starch indicator.

2. To make the dilute solution needed in this unit, mix 10 ml (⅓ oz) of tincture of iodine with 240 ml (approximately 8 oz) of water. Store the dilute solution in a dark bottle to prevent light from causing it to degrade.

Making Protein Test Papers (Coomassie Blue Papers)
Protein test papers may be purchased directly from Carolina Biological Supply Company. Alternatively, you can make your own.

To make the protein test papers yourself

1. Order Coomassie blue powder (catalog no. 97-2981) from Carolina Biological Supply Company.

2. Dissolve 5 grams of the powder in 100 ml of a solution consisting of 10 ml 1 Normal acetic acid, 40 ml methanol, and 50 ml water. This is a 5% solution of Coomassie blue.

3. Use the 5% Coomassie blue solution to make about 30 ml (1 oz) of a .05% Coomassie blue solution. To do so, put about seven drops of the 5% solution in 30 ml (1 oz) of developer solution, a 1-to-100 dilution. See Lesson 12, pg. 121, for information on making the developer solution.

4. Use either white filter paper or 300-inch rolls of Whatman #1 chromatography paper to make the test strips. Cut the paper into strips about 15 cm (6") long and about 4 cm (1½") wide.

5. In a petri dish or any flat dish, pour a thin layer (just covering the bottom) of the .05% Coomassie blue solution.

APPENDIX C

6. Dip the long edge of the paper into the solution so that approximately 6 mm (¼") of the edge of the paper is blue (see Figure C-1). Dry the papers overnight.

7. Cut the paper into strips approximately 1 cm (⅜") wide.

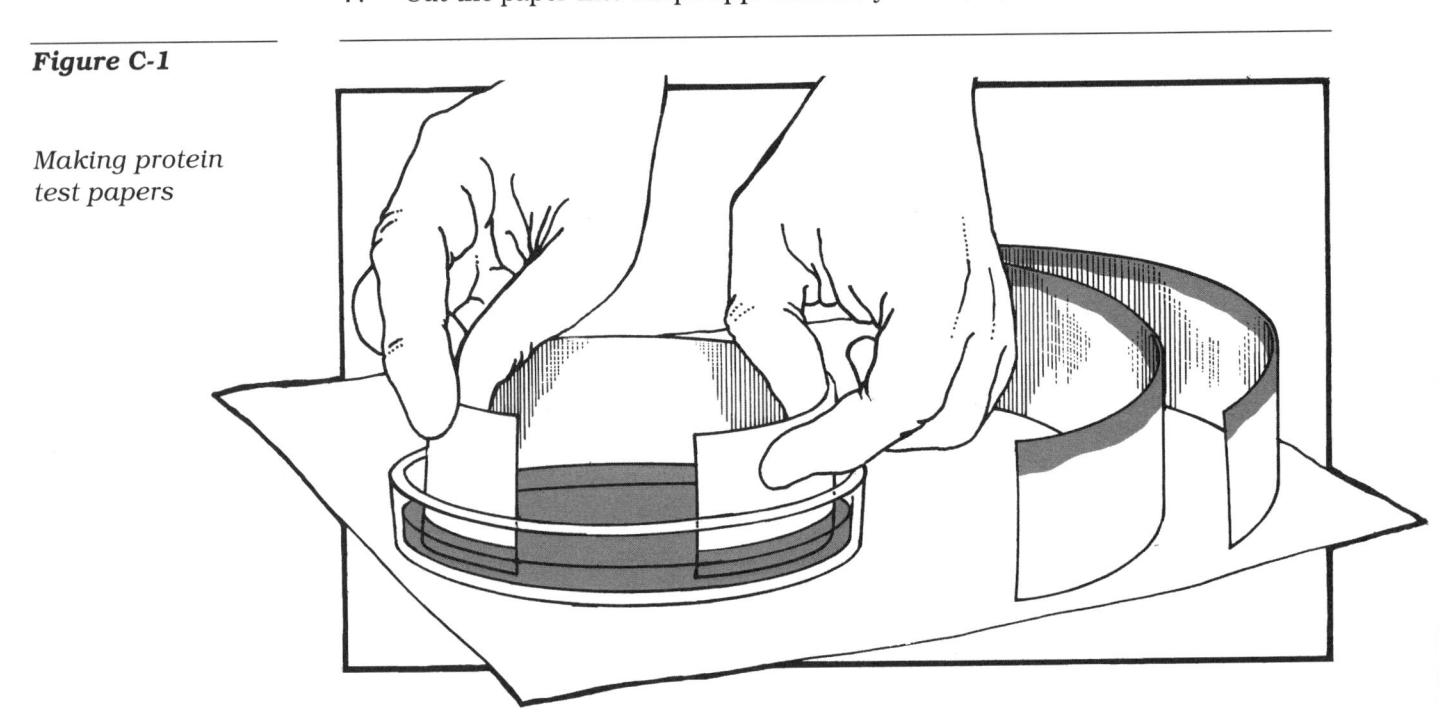

Figure C-1

Making protein test papers

180 / Making Test Solutions and Papers STC / *Food Chemistry*

APPENDIX D

Dietary Guidelines

Dietary guidelines have been established by a variety of cooperating federal agencies, including the U.S. Department of Agriculture (USDA) and the U.S. Department of Health and Human Services (HHS). The Food Guide Pyramid illustration on the next page presents a general guide for meeting dietary recommendations. Consumers can use the illustration and other publications from the USDA and HHS as guidelines for eating in ways that meet dietary recommendations. There are differences among documents with recommendations in the way foods are grouped (e.g., where legumes are placed) and in how many servings are recommended from each group (e.g., should both vegetables and fruits have a minimum recommended number of servings?). Nevertheless, these recommendations are very similar in the general eating patterns they put forth.

APPENDIX D

Food Guide Pyramid

A Guide to Daily Food Choices

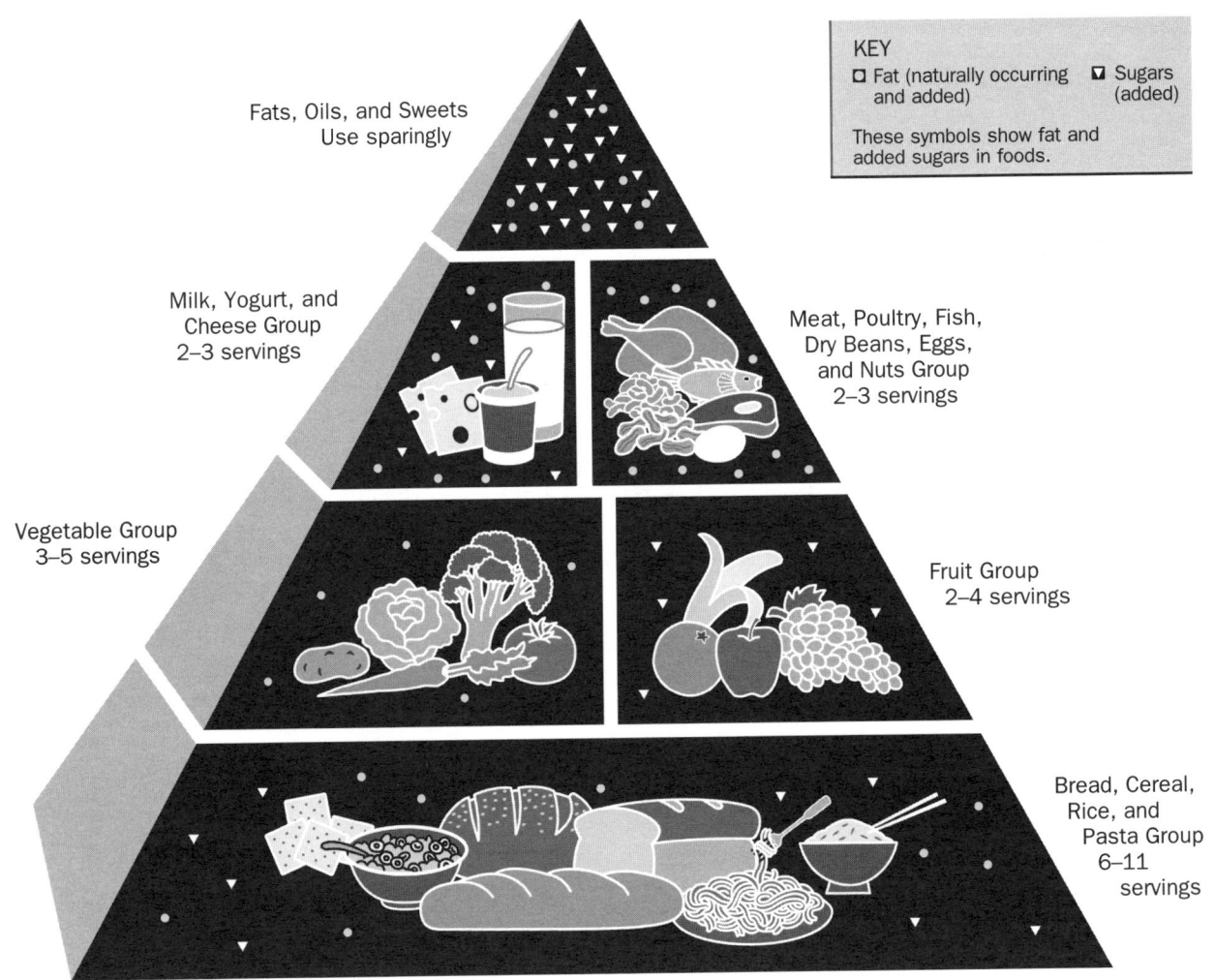

KEY
- ☐ Fat (naturally occurring and added)
- ▼ Sugars (added)

These symbols show fat and added sugars in foods.

Fats, Oils, and Sweets
Use sparingly

Milk, Yogurt, and Cheese Group
2–3 servings

Meat, Poultry, Fish, Dry Beans, Eggs, and Nuts Group
2–3 servings

Vegetable Group
3–5 servings

Fruit Group
2–4 servings

Bread, Cereal, Rice, and Pasta Group
6–11 servings

SOURCE: U.S. Department of Agriculture/U.S. Department of Health and Human Services

National Science Resources Center Advisory Board

Chair

S. Anders Hedberg, Director, Science Education Initiatives, Bristol-Myers Squibb Foundation, Princeton, N.J.

Members

Gaurdie E. Banister, President, Shell Services International, Inc., Houston, Tex.

Ann Bay, Associate Director, George Washington's Mount Vernon Estate and Gardens, Mount Vernon, Va.

Goéry Delacôte, Executive Director, The Exploratorium, San Francisco, Calif.

Peter Dow, President, First-Hand Learning, Inc., Buffalo, N.Y.

Joyce Dutcher, Project Manager, Houston Urban Learning Initiative, Houston Independent School District, Houston, Tex.

Hubert M. Dyasi, Director, The Workshop Center, City College School of Education (The City University of New York), New York, N.Y.

Sylvia A. Earle, Director, Chair, and Founder, DOER Marine Operation, Oakland, Calif.

Guillermo Fernández de la Garza, Executive Director, United States-Mexico Foundation for Science, Mexico City, Mexico

Bernard S. Finn, Curator, Division of Electricity and Modern Physics, National Museum of American History, Smithsonian Institution, Washington, D.C.

Elsa Garmire, Professor, Thayer School of Engineering, Dartmouth College, Hanover, N.H.

Richard M. Gross, Vice President and Director, Research and Development, The Dow Chemical Company, Midland, Mich.

Richard Hinman, Senior Vice President for Research and Development (retired), Central Research Division, Pfizer Inc., Groton, Conn.

David Jenkins, Associate Director for Interpretive Programs, National Zoological Park, Smithsonian Institution, Washington, D.C.

John W. Layman, Professor Emeritus of Education and Physics, University of Maryland, College Park, Md.

Leon M. Lederman, Nobel Laureate, Resident Scholar, Illinois Mathematics and Science Academy, Aurora, Ill., and Director Emeritus, Fermi National Accelerator Laboratory, Batavia, Ill.

Thomas T. Liao, Professor and Chair, Department of Technology and Society, and Director, Professional Education Program, College of Engineering and Applied Sciences, State University of New York, Stony Brook, N.Y.

Theodore A. Maxwell, Associate Director, Collections and Research, National Air and Space Museum, Smithsonian Institution, Washington, D.C.

Mara Mayor, Director, The Smithsonian Associates, Smithsonian Institution, Washington, D.C.

Joseph A. Miller, Jr., Senior Vice President, Research and Development, and Chief Technology Officer, E.I. du Pont de Nemours & Company, Wilmington, Del.

John A. Moore, Professor Emeritus, Department of Biology, University of California, Riverside, Calif.

Cherry A. Murray, Director of Physical Sciences, Bell Labs, Lucent Technologies, Murray Hill, N.J.

Carlo Parravano, Director, The Merck Institute for Science Education, Rahway, N.J.

Robert W. Ridky, Professor, Department of Geology, University of Maryland, College Park, Md.

Robert D. Sullivan, Associate Director for Public Programs, National Museum of Natural History, Smithsonian Institution, Washington, D.C.

Gerald F. Wheeler, Executive Director, National Science Teachers Association, Arlington, Va.

Meredith Harris Willcuts, Science Coordinator/Science Specialist, Walla Walla School District, Walla Walla, Wash.

Paul H. Williams, Emeritus Professor, Wisconsin Fast Plants Program, University of Wisconsin, Madison, Wis.

Karen L. Worth, Senior Associate, Urban Elementary Science Project, Education Development Center, Newton, Mass.

Ex Officio Members

E. William Colglazier, Executive Officer, National Academy of Sciences, Washington, D.C.

Michael Feuer, Executive Director, Center for Science, Mathematics, and Engineering Education, National Research Council, Washington, D.C.

J. Dennis O'Connor, Under Secretary for Science, Smithsonian Institution, Washington, D.C.

Mary Tanner, Senior Executive Officer, Office of the Under Secretary for Science, Smithsonian Institution, Washington, D.C.